Medical Statistics on Microcomputers

A guide to the appropriate use of statistical packages

MEDICAL STATISTICS ON MICRO-COMPUTERS

A guide to the appropriate use of statistical packages

R A Brown
Department of Mathematics and Computer Science,
University of Dundee
and
J Swanson Beck
Department of Pathology,
Ninewells Hospital and Medical School,
Dundee

Articles reprinted from the *Journal of Clinical Pathology*
Published by the British Medical Journal
Tavistock Square, London WC1H 9JR

First published December 1990

British Library Cataloguing in Publication Data
Brown, R. A.
Medical statistics on microcomputers.
1. Medicine. Statistics
I. Title   II. Beck, J. Swanson
610.21

ISBN 0–7279–0290–3

Printed in Great Britain by
Latimer Trend & Company Ltd, Plymouth

Contents

	Page
Introduction	ix
Data handling	1
Summarising data	11
Analysis of data from one or two groups: Confidence intervals and significance tests	20
Comparison of several groups: The analysis of variance	34
Analysis of continuous data that is not normally distributed: Distribution free methods	43
Are variables related? Correlation and regression	52
Analysis of categorical data	70
Statistical methods for diagnostic tests	87
Index	101

Introduction

Recent developments in microcomputer technology, particularly the introduction of the IBM personal computer and the mass production of inexpensive "clones", have put within reach of the budgets of most laboratories relatively powerful machines such as the XT and AT models. In response to growing demand computer software has been written to perform a wide range of tasks, and very sophisticated programs are now available at modest prices. Consequently, most workers in pathology laboratories are likely to have access to computer power that could not have been imagined a decade ago. As a result the users of statistical techniques need no longer be concerned with the arithmetical and algebraic details of various statistical methods and can concentrate instead on understanding the underlying ideas and basic principles of statistical analysis.

This book has been written to show how microcomputers can be used to facilitate the analysis of data. It is our intention:

(i) to explain the rational basis of widely applicable statistical methods without requiring the reader to understand the underlying algebra; and

(ii) to summarise the limitations of the various statistical procedures so that the user can make an informed choice when analysing data.

We do not intend to present an extensive account of the design of clinical trials as the techniques and approaches applicable to this type of work have recently been discussed fairly exhaustively.[1,2] We shall concentrate, instead, on statistical methods applicable to most laboratory investigations. Details of the algebraic formulae used for particular statistical methods may be obtained from standard texts.[3-5]

1

Data handling

Organisation of information in the microcomputer

In certain specialised applications data are transferred directly from analytical apparatus to a microcomputer via a connecting cable. Diverse observations made on each individual patient or specimen, however, will more commonly be keyed in manually before any statistical analysis can be done. The microcomputer can store data in files on a floppy or hard disc, depending on the configuration of the machine. The way in which files are stored need not concern us here as the disc operating system (DOS) takes care of this.

To put the data into the file system the user has three options: the data can be entered by using (a) a proprietary Spreadsheet program, (b) a proprietary Database Management System (DBMS), or (c) the data entry facilities within the statistical analysis package.

Spreadsheets were invented in the 1970s to assist business people in making financial calculations, but they were very quickly adopted in areas of application which had nothing to do with finance. In financial calculations you usually have several columns of figures—for example, unit prices and quantities of goods ordered—and you want to make up an invoice, say, which involves calculating the actual price for each invoiced item by multiplying quantity ordered by unit price. These figures will need to be placed in a third column. If value added tax (or local sales tax) has to be added then a further calculation is required, the values in the actual price column must be multiplied by the appropriate tax rate, and the results must be placed in a fourth column. The price charged will be the sum of these two columns and this will need to be displayed as a fifth column. Finally, these columns must be added up to give the total price excluding tax, the total tax, and the total price including tax.

Anyone who has struggled with the data resulting from a biomedical investigation will recognise that the types of calculation involved in preparing an invoice, adding columns together, taking a percentage of each value in a column and so on, are familiar operations. Hence the widespread adoption of spreadsheets as aids to data manipulation outside the financial world. There are several professionally produced spreadsheet programs on the market, any computer magazine will list perhaps a dozen or more. One of the market leaders is called Lotus 1-2-3, others are Supercalc and VP Planner, but Lotus 1-2-3 has more or less set the standard in this field and has sold more than half a million copies. All spreadsheets work in essentially the same way, but the user must check that the spreadsheet they have chosen stores data on file in a manner compatible with the statistical package they intend to use.

Spreadsheet programs are incredibly easy to use. Initially the user is presented with a blank screen organised into columns. Each row can therefore represent a subject and each column the value of a particular type of observation. Data may be typed from the computer keyboard into any row or column. There is also a special facility for defining the values which are to go into a particular column in terms of the values present in other columns. For instance, you might wish to give an instruction such as "make each value in column 3 equal to the corresponding value in column 1 minus the corresponding value in column 2". Once such an instruction has been given the spreadsheet program will automatically calculate these values, and what is more it will store this definition as part of the spreadsheet data file. This means that if the user subsequently changes any of the values in columns 1 or 2 the corresponding changes to column 3 will occur automatically. This is an example of the use of a very simple arithmetic expression, but all sorts of much more complicated column definitions are available; you could, if you wished, define column 5 in a particular spreadsheet as the logarithm of the squares of the values in columns 1 and 2 divided by the square root of the ratio of the values in columns 3 and 4.

There are also special commands for entering repetitive values into a column. For example, data may be gathered on 300 subjects, of whom 120 are healthy controls, 105 are patients with pulmonary tuberculosis and 75 are patients with leprosy. To distinguish the three groups it is customary to use codes such as $1 = $ normal, $2 = $ pulmonary tuberculosis, and $3 = $ leprosy, so that one variable in the data file should consist of 120 ones, followed by 105 twos, and then 75 threes. The spreadsheet program has special facilities for defining a column consisting of 120 ones, 105 twos, and 75 threes in that order, so that the user is relieved of the drudgery of typing in all this repetitive information.

Databases The spreadsheet can be seen as the electronic equivalent of a large table. An alternative manual system of record keeping is to have a record card for each individual with labelled spaces for the data. This results in a stack of record cards rather than a table: the computer implementation of this is a DBMS. The user designs a master form which contains blank spaces for the data and this is stored on disc. To facilitate data entry it is a good idea to make the screen format look like the corresponding manual record card. To store a series of records the DBMS presents the user with a fresh pro-forma on screen for each record: each item can then be inserted into the appropriate blank space. This method is preferable when a large number of records have to be filed; the use of the master as a prompt to the user greatly reduces the incidence of errors.

Good statistical packages have data entry facilities which usually operate on something like the spreadsheet principle so it is not essential to use one of the spreadsheet or DBMS programs, but many workers find such programs convenient. It must be emphasised, however, that individual data management systems may store data on disc in different formats. If a proprietary program is used then care must be taken to ensure that the format is compatible with that of the statistical package.

The method is very simple in Statgraphics. The first procedure in transferring a file from a spreadsheet in Lotus 1-2-3 is to introduce a temporary change to the "System Profile" to ensure that the import pathway is switched to the appropriate Lotus file on the hard disc. The "Import" menu is then called up, import file type is given as Lotus, the original ".WKS" file name is entered and the new Statgraphics file name specified; after pressing the "F6" key the transfer will be accomplished automatically.

VARIABILITY

If there were no variability in results there would not be any need for statistical analysis to aid in the interpretation of data from experiments or clinical observation. We all appreciate that variability in our results is often great and we optimistically resort to statistical analysis for support or guidance. There is no single cause of variability, which can arise from three main sources.

(1) Methodology All methods of measurement give results that are estimates of the underlying absolute value. Those which are based on direct physical measurement, such as length, weight, or temperature, are usually relatively accurate, provided the apparatus is functioning properly and no errors are introduced in recording, but it is clear that the more indirect the measurement process the greater the variability that will arise. When a metabolic activity is assessed by use of a radioactive tracer, the counts that result will be subject to Poisson variability arising from the intermittent process of atomic disintegration. Even greater variability may arise if some form of interpolation or mathematical modelling is required to interpret the experimental results. An important distinction must be remembered: *accuracy* is an indication of how close the measurement will be to the absolute value; *precision* is a measure of how close replicates will be to each other. High precision will arise from good technical work, but it does not necessarily indicate good accuracy. Precision can, in principle, be measured quite easily as all that has to be done is to compare a series of replicate measurements. Accuracy is much more difficult to ascertain as the replicate measurements of a known standard must be compared. This standard has to be specially prepared and you must be sure that its value is actually known and that it does not deteriorate with time.

(2) Sampling Because it is not usually practicable to measure all the material in a specimen and it is certainly not possible to measure all relevant aspects of a patient, there will inevitably be variability inherent in the actual part of the sample that is being analysed. Sometimes this will not be great—for example, one aliquot from a serum sample is unlikely to differ widely from another, provided deterioration has not occurred in the intervening time—but whenever tissue samples, cells, or particles are involved there is considerable potential for variation among samples (even serial histological sections can vary considerably from each other), and greater differences may be seen between different biopsy specimens when the underlying disease is focal.

(3) Human variation Even in healthy subjects there can be variation, reflecting different genetic backgrounds or biological

experience. Moreover, there can be variations with time due to oscillations of physiological behaviour that may or may not be in phase with an easily recognisable periodicity, such as diurnal rhythm. There are even greater sources of variation in patients in whom severity of disease or response to treatment differs.

In the planning of any investigation it is essential that care is taken to minimise controllable sources of variability and to recognise the aspects that are beyond the control of the investigator. In this way the investigator optimises the chance of getting data which can be analysed successfully. It must always be remembered that the basic purpose of an investigation is not to accumulate numbers and to be busy, but rather to draw conclusions from a particular study that can legitimately be applied throughout the world to improve understanding of biomedical mechanisms, or the natural history of disease, and to provide the basis for better treatment of patients in clinical practice.

TYPES OF INVESTIGATION

Statisticians distinguish between experimental investigations and observational studies, and the distinction is important as there are more problems with the interpretation of the results of a statistical analysis applied to the latter. *Experimental investigations* aim to compare two or more *treatments*, such as the administration of various drugs, applied to groups of subjects, or to investigate the consequences of deliberate variation of *factors* which are controlled by the investigator. A typical example of a study of this type would be the investigation of the effect of storage temperature on the recovery of bone marrow cells for transplantation. The sample of bone marrow was split into aliquots each of which was stored at one of a number of predetermined temperatures, and the viability of the cells was measured at the end of the fixed in vitro storage periods. The aliquots to be stored at each temperature were chosen at random, and identical methods were used to measure viability in all samples so that the effect of other variables was minimised.

In an experimental investigation the investigator has complete freedom to decide which experimental subject should be assigned to each treatment. There will inevitably be unsuspected differences between people even within a homogeneous group, and to ensure that these are evened out and so do not bias observed mean responses it is essential to allocate patients randomly to the treatment groups. This process is known as *randomisation* and it

5

ensures the validity of the interference that observed differences between groups are caused by the different treatment they have received.

In summary, an experimental investigation entails the following:
(i) *replication*, several patients or units of experimental material allocated to each group;
(ii) allocation of subjects to treatments under the control of the investigator;
(iii) randomisation.

In contrast, an *observational study* usually lacks the second and third elements listed above. For example, an observational study of the prognostic value of microscopical and other features of primary tumours in breast cancer might proceed by extracting all available case records and specimens. Measurements or gradings of potentially important characteristics, such as tumour size, and of other possible prognostic indicators, such as the extent of lymph node disease, would be recorded. The investigator might then divide the cases into two groups—poor and good survival—and look for some subset of the recorded features, a discriminating subset, which differs substantially between the two groups. Once this has been found, one can combine the values of several features in the discriminating subset to yield a score for each patient, and this is used as a predictor of survival in new cases. Note that the composition of the groups is not, and cannot be, controlled by the investigator as it is clearly impossible to allocate patients randomly to the poor and good survival groups. Consequently, considerable caution must be exercised in ascribing the observed differences among the prognostic features to the overt difference between survival experience. There could well be some unsuspected factors which were seriously unbalanced between the two groups that could equally well be the explanation of the observed differences. It is therefore essential to verify the results of potentially important observational studies by the accumulation of further data in follow up studies in which the discriminating criteria are applied to new cases.

Statistical packages for microcomputers

There are several good quality statistical packages available which, when used in a knowledgeable way, allow the experimenter to use many more methods than is practical using traditional paper calculations. This book will be illustrated by reference to the working of two well known packages—Minitab and Statgraphics. These packages have a good reputation in the field of statistics and have been evaluated by bodies such as the American Statistical Association, which runs a continuing programme of package review and evaluation. Both have clearly written, unambiguous manuals. There are other less expensive packages but we have not used them; the principles that we explain in this book should be generally applicable.

The data can be entered directly into the statistical package from the keyboard, or indirectly from a spreadsheet or a database. Statgraphics uses a spreadsheet format for the entry of data. Data are stored as variables, each occupying a column, and these variables are in turn organised into files. The files are stored on the hard disc. Each variable has to be given a name by the user, the naming convention is quite flexible, up to 10 alpha numeric characters may be used to make up a variable name, the only restriction being that the name must begin with a letter. Thus "age", "sex", "wbc" and "OKT4" are all valid names but "3-HTdR" is not as it begins with a numeral and contains a hyphen. Each file must also be given a name by the user with a similar flexibility in the naming convention, up to eight alpha numeric characters are allowed, beginning with a letter. Hence "lymphoma", "Crohns" and "Hodgkins" are valid file names but "Crohn's" is not as it contains an apostrophe.

To make it easy to see what is stored on the hard disc Statgraphics creates a "data directory" at the start of each session. This is a complete list of all the Statgraphics data files and the variables stored in them. By moving a cursor to any desired variable it is possible to display its contents, get a printed copy of it, or insert it as the name of a variable within a Statgraphics procedure.

To create a new file containing several variables you select the "Data Management" option from the main menu. After selection of the relevant options from two submenus you are faced with a spreadsheet display into which you can insert the names of variables (as column headings) and enter the values of these variables from the keyboard. This is done using the Statgraphics "full screen editor", a subprogram designed to make data entry or editing of Statgraphics data files particularly easy. Once the file is complete, or indeed at any intermediate stage, it can be saved on to disc. If a file is particularly long the user may wish to create it over several Statgraphics sessions, adding further data to the file at each session.

Thereafter the statistical package is driven by the operator selecting a procedure from a menu (fig 1) or by a system of brief but memorable commands, whichever is appropriate to the design of the package or the convenience of the user. At various points in certain analyses, the user is allowed to select from a range of options to see plots or perform supplementary analyses. All of the common methods of display, summary, and analysis are literally at the user's fingertips, but current statistical packages, being essentially "unintelligent", are incapable of advising on the most appropriate method for a particular data set and this remains the prerogative of the user.

The statistical packages arrange the data in spreadsheet form so it is important to identify variables unambiguously and to identify missing values. The conventions of the package must be rigidly adhered to if malfunction is to be avoided.

STATGRAPHICS *statistical graphics system*

DATA MANAGEMENT AND SYSTEM UTILITIES
- A.   Data Management
- B.   System Environment
- C.   Report Writer and Graphics Replay
- D.   Plotter Interface

PLOTTING AND DESCRIPTIVE STATISTICS
- E.   Plotting Functions
- F.   Descriptive Methods
- G.   Estimation and Testing
- H.   Distribution Functions
- I.   Exploratory Data Analysis

ANOVA AND REGRESSION ANALYSIS
- J.   Analysis of Variance
- K.   Regression Analysis

TIME SERIES PROCEDURES
- L.   Forecasting
- M.   Quality Control
- N.   Smoothing
- O.   Time Series Analysis

ADVANCED PROCEDURES
- P.   Categorical Data Analysis
- Q.   Multivariate Methods
- R.   Nonparametric Methods
- S.   Sampling
- T.   Experimental Design

MATHEMATICAL AND USER PROCEDURES
- U.   Mathematical Functions
- V.   Supplementary Operations

Use cursor keys to highlight desired section. Then press ENTER.

Figure 1   The Statgraphics main menu allows the user to choose from a wide range of options.

Types of data

Data obtained by observation or measurement in the laboratory or clinic can be of three different types which must be distinguished clearly as different methods of analysis are appropriate for the various types of data.

Nominal data—the observations are classified into categories that are different in character and cannot be measured or ordered—for example, hair colour or race—often the named character can be only present ($+$) or absent ($-$).

Ordinal data—here the observations refer to a common character and they can be grouped into a limited number of categories which can be ordered in an ascending series or rank, such as staging of cancer: commonly such data are presented as $+$, $++$, or $+++$, but numbers can also be used to describe the categories so that there is a danger of confusion of this form of ranking with true measurements. It is essential to remember that in ordinal data the grouping is only semiquantitative and that $+$ is not half as big as $++$: moreover, the intervals between successive categories will probably be different.

Continuous data—is the term used to describe observations made on a scale which has a natural zero and a well defined unit of measurement, such as length: the observations will usually be expressed as decimal numbers.

Both nominal and ordinal data give rise to counts of the frequency of occurrence of the various categories within the groups of subjects under investigation and these counts are naturally whole numbers. They may be converted into rates, proportions, or percentages; when expressed in this form they appear to be decimal numbers but they are essentially different in character from continuous data and need appropriately different statistical treatment.

Appendix

MISSING VALUES

If certain observations are not available then this must be indicated during data entry by using a "missing value code" to represent them. In Statgraphics a missing value is indicated by leaving a blank in the corresponding position in the worksheet; in Minitab an asterisk is used instead of a blank.

When the experimenter is aware that there are missing data the manual for the package should be consulted to verify if there is some method of specifying missing values, otherwise every analysis will have to be preceded by a data editing session to weed out the cases with missing values—a very tedious business.

IMPORTING SPREADSHEET AND DATABASE FILES

Importing is the name given to the process for transferring data files from proprietary spreadsheets and DBMS into a statistical package. Statgraphics will cope with files from Lotus 1-2-3, Symphony, and dBase III. Minitab can read files from Lotus 1-2-3 only, but certain "Lotus-clones" may be acceptable.

COMMAND LINES

The Minitab package uses commands in preference to a menu system; the user specifies the task to be done by typing a command line. Minitab uses command lines which are reasonably memorable—for example, the sequence of commands:

> NAME C1 'height'
> NAME C2 'weight'
> DOTPLOT 'height'
> PLOT 'height' vs 'weight'

names the first and second columns of the worksheet height and weight and produces a dotplot of height and a plot of height against weight.

2

Summarising data

Data displays and statistical summaries

It is important that any conclusion to be drawn from an experiment is intuitively acceptable as "common sense" and that statistical methods are used to facilitate objective assessment of results. It is therefore essential that the experimenter examines the "raw" data from every experiment. Graphical displays have an immediate visual impact and a compactness that is always absent from numerical tables. Differences between groups, variability within groups, time trends, or other forms of associations between sets of measurements can be investigated and communicated by simple well designed graphical displays. Such displays are a valuable feature of all good statistical packages—Statgraphics is particularly good in this respect. There are no rigid rules for the selection of the most appropriate method of display to show the magnitude and variability of the observations in any particular experiment. The choice is guided by informed common sense, but the chosen format should, in the first instance, present all the original observations (not just condensed summaries) to allow the observer to "eyeball" the results and judge the plausibility of any conclusions presented.

A basic assumption of several widely used statistical methods is that the groups of results being compared have similar variability and this can often be assessed by visual inspection of their distributions. Such preliminary examination of the data can usually be performed conveniently on the visual display screen of the microcomputer. When the data sets are large some summarised form of display may be needed because of the confusion of overlapping points on the screen, but, whatever the method, it must present a fair and unbiased view of the variability of the data.

The dot plot—All the observations are displayed by symbols in a vertical array alongside an appropriate scale (fig 2A). This plot gives a visual indication of the magnitude and spread of each set of values, but comparisons of sets of values are more difficult than they appear: it is therefore useful to supplement the display with indicators of the group means at least.

The histogram is an alternative display that is useful when each group consists of a large number of measurements (100 or more). The interval of the measurement scale which contains all the data is divided into equal subintervals and the number of values falling into each subinterval is represented by a rectangle with height proportional to this number. Care is needed in the selection of the subintervals as too many will reduce the number of values in each one, emphasising minor fluctuation, and too few will obscure the true variability of the data. The Statgraphics package is capable of generating histogram displays automatically but the user can easily choose a preferred style that overrides the inbuilt criteria for selection of interval size.

The fact that the individual observations are not shown and that the number of intervals is chosen subjectively makes this a poor choice for final presentation of results. Because of this, many scientific journals have a policy of not publishing data in histogram format.

SUMMARY STATISTICS TO INDICATE LOCATION, SPREAD, AND SYMMETRY

There are a few simple statistics that can convey a lot of information about a set of observations. Most standard statistical methods for analysing two or more sets of measurements assume that:

(1) each set has more or less the same variability;

(ii) the distribution of values around the mean is more or less symmetrical (for "parametric" analyses), or has a similar shape in each group;

(iii) there are no outliers (values far removed from the main body) in the data.

Magnitude An indication of the "middle" of the data gives useful information when attempting to determine whether groups of data are similar or different. Two statistics commonly used for this purpose are the *mean* (arithmetical average) and the *median* (middle value when the observations are ranked in order). Either value will be equally informative when the distribution is symmetrical but the mean forms the basis of certain standard methods for assessing differences between groups. If the mean and the median are quite different this indicates serious asymmetry, and methods of statistical analysis based on medians and on rank order of data will be necessary (details are given in later chapters of this book). Outliers do not affect the median but they may make the mean unrepresentative.

Spread—Again there is a choice of summary statistics. The *standard deviation* (SD) is widely used, but it is valid only when the data are more or less symmetrical: it is the square root of the average of the squared deviations of the data values from the mean. An alternative is the *interquartile range* (fig 2B): when the data are ordered the upper and lower quartiles are the values that separate off the upper and lower 25% of the values; thus the interquartile range measures the middle 50% of the data and this is valid whether or not the data are symmetrically distributed. The *range*— the difference between the largest and smallest values—is much less informative because it is so sensitive to outliers. All these summary statistics are readily generated in microcomputer packages.

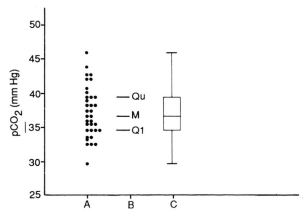

Figure 2   Various displays of transcutaneous measurements of pCO_2 in forearm skin of normal subjects. (A) A dot plot of the data. (B) The interquartile range spans the central 50% of the data. (C) The box and whisker plot suppresses details but indicates spread and symmetry.

13

Symmetry This can be assessed from a "box and whisker plot" which indicates graphically the median, quartiles, and range of a set of data and can easily be generated in both packages (fig 2C). The central 50% of the data is represented by a rectangle extending from the lower to the upper quartile, the median being indicated by a bar across the rectangle. The "whiskers" extend to the extremes unless there are values which are far away from the central 50% (outliers), in which case the length of the corresponding whisker is set at one and a half times the interquartile range, and the outlying points are plotted individually.

Sometimes asymmetrical data sets can be converted into a more or less symmetrical form by *"transformation"* of the raw results by taking logarithms, square roots, or other simple mathematical functions (fig 3), and such procedures can be performed automatically with most packages. Care should be taken if any values are less than zero because logarithms or square roots of negative numbers do not exist. Most packages will insert a "missing value code" in place of an impossible value when transforming; care should be taken to ascertain that the data are not unwittingly corrupted. A useful device is to add a suitable number to all observations to remove negative numbers. Transformation of data is a useful approach; if it is successful it permits the use of statistical methods which require symmetrical distributions on data that are clearly asymmetrical in their raw form. Care is of course necessary when interpretating analyses performed on transformed data; in particular, it is necessary to "back transform" the values resulting from statistical analysis—for example, mean, confidence intervals, etc.—before attempting a biological or clinical interpretation of the outcome of the analysis.

DISPLAYS TO BE AVOIDED

One of the commonest forms of data presentation seen in articles published in biomedical journals is the "mean and error bar" plot. Here the original data are not shown, but the mean of each set is plotted with two equal bars above and below (fig 4). This type of plot has little to recommend it: it is misleading in several ways.

Firstly, the number of observations in each category is not clearly apparent and so disparity between size of groups being compared or the presence of a very small group that may not be representative can be obscured.

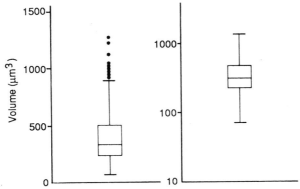

Figure 3   *(A) Box and whisker plot of volumes of 300 lymphocytes. The distribution is noticeably asymmetrical: in this situation the package calculates the length of the upper whisker as one and a half times the interquartile range (length of rectangle) and the outlying points are plotted individually (see text). (B) Box and whisker plot of the logarithms of the same data: the transformation has made the distribution symmetrical.*

Secondly, the presentation of the equal sized error bars above and below the mean can imply that the data are symmetrically distributed, but the reader cannot assess this for him/herself.

Thirdly, the basis of the calculation of the length of the error bars may be misleading because the indicated range will contain only about 70% of the observations if the standard deviation is

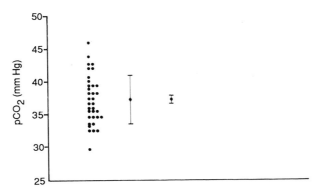

Figure 4   *Transcutaneous measurement of pCO_2. The mean and error bar plot (larger bars) understates the variability: using the SEM (smaller bars) gives a very misleading impression of variability.*

chosen. Choice of the standard error of the mean (SEM)—SD divided by square root of number of observations—to indicate variability is even more misleading as the real extent of variability will be seriously understated, particularly for large samples.

It is clearly not very sensible to replace sets of two or three observations by their mean and standard deviation as the actual values could just as easily be presented and would more clearly tell the story.

OUTLIERS

Occasional values that are considerably larger or smaller than the main group are termed *outliers*. Such observations are commoner than is popularly supposed, but they will be unlikely to be appreciated unless the data are displayed using either a dot or box and whisker plot format. Sometimes an outlier is an artefact due to an error in transcription or instrument reading, sometimes it has resulted from inclusion of a result that is inappropriate—for example, erroneous selection of a patient or misclassification of an observation. It is good practice to check the validity of outlier observations, but each observation must be accepted unless there is clear evidence that it is artefactual.

Most of the standard methods that use means and standard deviations are adversely affected by the presence of outliers. Methods which use medians, quartiles, and ranks are generally much less vulnerable to distortion by outliers. It is not possible to give guidelines on how to deal with outliers. Perhaps the safest policy is to be constantly aware of the potential hazards and when outliers are encountered to analyse the data with and without the inclusion of the suspect values. When the results remain substantially unchanged, then you can be reassured that the conclusions drawn from the statistical analysis have not been unduly influenced by the outlier values. When the analyses disagree, however, it is obvious that the outlier values are influencing the analysis. In this situation advice should be sought from a professional statistician who may advise the use of a more valid method of analysis with statistical procedures that are less influenced by outliers.

THE NORMAL DISTRIBUTION

Many standard statistical analyses of continuous data are based on the assumption that the spread of values across the population can be described by the so-called "normal" distribution. This form of distribution was originally selected as the basis of much statistical work because it is unimodal and symmetrical, with a high proportion of values relatively close to the mean and decreasing concentration of values in the "tails" of the distribution, similar to many distributions observed in practice. It is undoubtedly a convenient approximation for many sets of data, but it would be wrong to assume that this particular distribution was a biologically "natural" pattern to which all "good" data conform—for example, the distribution of survival times of patients with cancer is not well approximated by the normal distribution.

The normal distribution curve illustrates the way in which a measurement might be expected to vary across a population (fig 5). The peak of the curve is located at the population mean and there is a precise relation between the population mean and standard deviation and the proportion of measurements lying within any specified range. For example, the statement that 95% of the values will be within 1·96 population standard deviations either side of the population mean is true for every normal distribution.

As normality is an important assumption for several statistical methods it is important to be able to assess whether a particular set

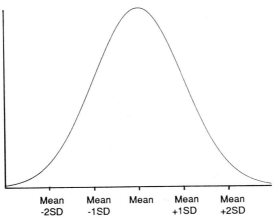

| Mean | Mean | Mean | Mean | Mean |
| -2SD | -1SD | | +1SD | +2SD |

Figure 5   The normal distribution is symmetrical and unimodal: the area under any portion of the curve indicates the probability that an observation will lie within the corresponding range—for example, 68% of observations will lie within 1 SD of the mean.

of data shows evidence of serious non-normality. The common methods of statistical analysis are fairly "robust to non-normality" provided that:

    (i) the data are more or less symmetrically distributed;

    (ii) the spread of results is similar in the groups being compared;

    (iii) there are no outliers in the data.

These methods can give rise to misleading results if these requirements are not met.

A simple graphical technique known as normal plotting may be used to assess normality. When performed manually the data values in a single sample are ordered and each value is plotted against the value you would expect to observe if the data were normally distributed. If the data are approximately normally distributed then the plotted points should show a straight line trend. The method is tedious to use manually but with suitable programs a normal plot can be displayed within minutes on a microcomputer. In Statgraphics the individual observations are displayed on an appropriate scale and the best fitting straight line is included so that visual assessment of departure from linearity can be made. If the data are effectively normally distributed the plotted

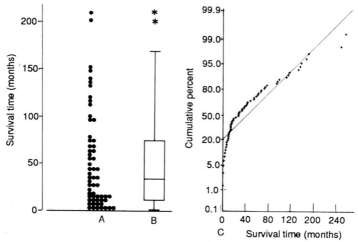

Figure 6   *Survival of 60 patients with breast cancer. (A) Dot plot indicates asymmetry; (B) box and whisker plot indicates that the upper 50% of the survival times are spread over a much greater range than the lower 50%; (C) normal plot shows pronounced curvature, hence the data distribution is very non-normal.*

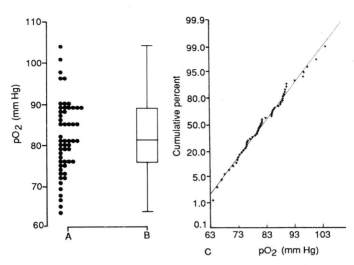

Figure 7   Transcutaneous measurements of pO₂ in forearm skin of 54 normal subjects. (A) Dot plot shows no pronounced asymmetry; (B) box and whisker plot clearly indicates near symmetry of the distribution; the median is more or less centrally placed, the whiskers are of almost equal length; (C) normal plot—no serious departure from normality.

points will be close to the fitted line, but will show pronounced deviations when the data are seriously non-normal.

To indicate how the method works in practice, consider the data on survival times of a group of patients with breast cancer, displayed as a dot plot in fig 6A, a box and whisker plot in fig 6B, and as a normal plot in fig 6C. Mean survival at 58·5 months is small compared with the sample standard deviation (45 months), which indicates possible asymmetry. The box and whisker plot confirms this, indicating serious asymmetry, and the normal plot, which shows considerable curvature, rules out the normal distribution as an adequate approximation to these data. For comparison, fig 7 shows the corresponding displays for a set of 60 normally distributed measurements (in this case the pO₂ in the normal forearm skin measured transcutaneously): the pattern of points shows no serious departure from the fitted line.

3

Analysis of data from one or two groups: Confidence intervals and significance tests

Populations and samples

The previous chapter described methods for displaying and summarising data. Usually this is not an end in itself, and research workers will wish to extend their conclusions from their samples or experiments to medical practice in general by statistical analysis. It is an essential precondition of valid statistical inference that the groups of subjects included in an investigation are selected randomly from the populations which are being compared, and its aim is to make statements about these global populations based on sample data.

One of the simplest forms of investigation is the comparison of measurements made on two well defined groups of individuals which differ in some clearly specified way—for example, medical treatment, pathological state. The subjects in each group must constitute a random sample from the corresponding population, and as far as practicable, the only major difference between the two groups should be the factor under investigation.

Before the start of an investigation it is essential to define clearly the populations to be sampled when the investigation is expected to result in recommendations of methods of treatment, diagnosis, or prognosis. Failing this, although it is still possible to carry through all stages of a statistical analysis, the final conclusions will be less valuable because they will refer to poorly defined populations. It is regrettable that many scientific reports of otherwise clearly described investigations lack unambiguous definition of criteria for group selection.

An entire population may be accessible at the time of data collection but cost precludes the measurement of every subject. In other situations, especially in disease of gradual onset, the observer can identify fully established disease, but even though he or she is aware of their presence he or she does not have the access or aptitude to identify subjects with presymptomatic defects, such as Alzheimer's disease. In either situation the investigator will make measurements on groups of individuals who have been selected randomly from the corresponding populations. Consequently, there must always be some uncertainty in any general conclusions concerning differences between the populations inferred from differences between the samples, and so the methods used to summarise the conclusions must be based on probability.

The kind of general statements which may be validly made often refer to population means, so it is essential to have a clear idea of what a population mean is and the use to which it can be put. For any specified measurement which could be made on every individual in a well defined population the population mean is just the value which would be obtained if each member of the population were measured and the mean of all the measurements was calculated. Because biomedical investigations invariably rely on samples to provide information it is clear that a population mean is something that can never be determined. Instead, you must rely on the information provided by the sample mean. As long as the sample is randomly selected from the population you may use the sample mean to estimate the population mean. The use of the word "estimate" serves to indicate that the sample mean cannot provide complete knowledge of the population mean, there will always be some uncertainty about the exact population mean value. How much uncertainty there will be depends on the size of the sample, in general large samples allow a population mean to be estimated more precisely than small ones.

Fortunately, it is never necessary to know the exact value of a population mean; a reasonably precise estimate will always suffice. For example, although it might be fairly interesting to know that the use of a particular technique would increase the yield of viable cells by 47·398% (population mean), an investigator would be quite satisfied with the information that the technique was likely to increase yield by between 45% and 50%, which is the kind of information we can expect to obtain from an investigation based on random sampling. If a closer estimate is required then the investigator merely has to increase the sample size.

If every individual in a population were to be measured we

would usually be aware of considerable variation among the measured values. The population standard deviation, which is just the standard deviation of all the values, would be one way of quantifying this variability. This is another quantity which we can never know in practice, but it is important to be able to estimate it.

For example, whether a particular diagnostic test will be useful for screening purposes will depend on the overlap between the values obtained for normal healthy members of the population and those who require treatment. Implicit in this is the idea of two populations, which may be referred to as the healthy population and the abnormal population. The extent of overlap of the distribution of measurements in the two populations depends both on the difference between the population means and on the relative sizes of the population standard deviations.

This is illustrated in fig 8 where the bell-shaped curves are meant to indicate the population distributions of the test results. The position of the peak of a curve indicates the population mean, and its breadth is related to the population standard deviation. Consider the vertical line in fig 8A, corresponding to a test result of 130 units. The area under the curve labelled "healthy" to the right of this line indicates the proportion of the healthy population who will have a test result above 130 units. In the same way the area under the curve labelled "abnormal" to the left of the vertical line indicates the proportion of abnormal subjects who will have a test result below 130 units. Both proportions are quite large, each being of the order of 30–40%. If the rather naive decision rule, "classify as healthy if the test result is 130 units or less and as abnormal if it is more than 130 units" is used, then it is quite clear that the rule is not going to perform very well. In the long run 30–40% of healthy subjects will be misclassified as abnormal and a similar proportion of abnormal subjects will be misclassified as healthy. By moving the decision point up the scale it is possible to reduce the proportion of healthy subjects who would be misclassified, but only at the cost of misclassifying more abnormal subjects.

There is no good solution in this situation; the population means are too close together and the population standard deviations are too large for there to be any prospect of obtaining a decision rule which misclassifies only a very small proportion of each population. Contrast this with the situation illustrated in fig 8B. Here the population means are exactly the same as those in fig 8A, because the peaks of the curves are in the same positions, but the popula-

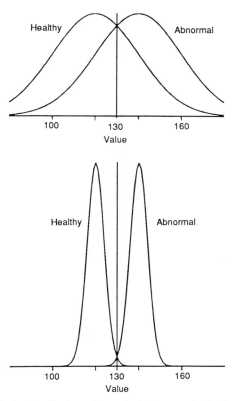

Figure 8 Population distributions of hypothetical test results for healthy and abnormal populations. (A) Separation is poor owing to large spread; (B) separation is almost perfect because spread is much smaller, even though population means are identical with (A).

tion standard deviations are much smaller and this results in the curves being much "slimmer". Now the same decision rule is very good at separating healthy subjects from abnormal ones; only a very small proportion of subjects will be misclassified.

Thus to evaluate a proposed quantitative diagnostic test it is necessary to have information about the relative separation of the population means and the sizes of the population standard deviations. Fortunately, it is not necessary to have exact information; estimates based on samples which are sufficiently large to provide a reasonable degree of precision will be adequate for all practical purposes. We hope that the reader will excuse the deliberate

23

vagueness here concerning what constitutes "sufficiently large" and "reasonable", this will be explained in chapter 8.

To summarise, the population mean and standard deviation are inaccessible, but they can be estimated by the *sample mean* and *sample standard deviation*, calculated from a random sample of members of the population. Statistical inference is concerned with:

(i)   making statements about population means or standard deviations, based on the limited information provided by the corresponding sample values;

(ii)   quantifying the uncertainty associated with these statements.

This enables statistical methods of various types to be used to assess whether for example, there is objective evidence for claiming that groups differ or that measurements are related. The practical application of this knowledge is the ability to determine whether groups of subjects differ in medically important ways or whether different types of measurements are related in ways which shed light on physiological, pathological, or biological mechanisms.

Estimating the population mean using a confidence interval

When a population is sampled, the sample mean is an estimate of the population mean. Other samples would produce different estimates and so it is important to be able to estimate the imprecision of an estimate from any given sample. Statisticians invented the term "confidence interval" to describe the range of plausible values for the population mean that are consistent with the observed sample mean.

Underlying the concept of the confidence interval is the realisation that the means of repeated samples will themselves have a distribution known as the *sampling distribution of the mean*. When the samples are selected from a normal population, the sampling distribution of the sample mean is normal with the same mean as the population, but with a standard deviation which is equal to the population standard deviation divided by the square root of the sample size. The standard deviation of the sampling distribution of the mean is called the "standard error of the mean" (SEM). Because the sampling distribution is normal, 95% of all sample means will lie within 1·96 SEM of the population mean. Given the actual value of the sample mean, the following argument produces the confidence interval for the population mean: suppose the observed sample mean is in fact one of the 95% that fall within 1·96 SEM of the population mean, then the population mean cannot be more than 1·96 SEM away from the sample mean. Consequently, the 95% confidence interval for the population mean is the range (sample mean − 1·96 SEM to sample mean + 1·96 SEM). We cannot be absolutely certain, however, that the sample mean is one of the 95% of sample means that are within 1·96 SEM of the population mean; there is a 5% chance that it is one of those that is not. So the statement "the population mean is within 1·96 SEM of the sample mean" will be correct 95 times out of 100, which is why the interval is called a 95% confidence interval. There is a minor technical difficulty as the SEM requires the population standard deviation value, which will be unknown in any practical situation. The sample standard deviation, however, can be used instead when calculating the SEM, with a correction to take into account the uncertainty arising from estimation of the population standard deviation by the sample standard deviation. This changes the number 1·96 to a somewhat larger value which depends on the sample size; it is 2·23 for samples of size 10, 2·09 for sample size 20, and 2·00 for samples of size 60 (values for all sample size may be obtained from a table of percentage points of the t-distribution.[6 12]).

Of course, there is no particular reason why the 95% probability level should be especially singled out; a higher value such as 99% might be preferable because then there is only one chance in 100 that the confidence interval fails to bracket the value of the population mean. By convention, the commonly used confidence intervals are 90%, 95%, and 99%. The higher the value selected for the probability that a given confidence level will include the population mean, the wider that interval will be. The point is illustrated as follows: 30 normal subjects were selected at random to estimate mean pO_2 in normal forearm skin, and the sample mean was 82·20 with a sample standard deviation of 8·97. Output from a Minitab analysis is shown in fig 9. The 95% confidence interval for the population mean $tcpO_2$ stretches from 78·85 up to 85·55; the corresponding 99% confidence interval is wider, stretching from 77·68 up to 86·71. The wider range of probable values for the population mean is the price which must be paid for being more confident that this range includes the population mean value.

MTB > describe, 'pO2'					
	N	MEAN	MEDIAN	TRMEAN	STDEV	SEMEAN
pO_2	30	82·20	82·38	82·05	8·97	1·64
	MIN	MAX	Q1	Q3		
pO_2	67·57	100·34	76·56	88·81		

MTB > TINTERVAL for, 'pO2'

	N	MEAN	STDEV	SE MEAN	95·0 PERCENT C.I.
pO_2	30	82·20	8·97	1·64	(78·85, 85·55)

MTB > TINTERVAL 99% for, 'pO2'

	N	MEAN	STDEV	SE MEAN	99·0 PERCENT C.I.
pO2	30	82·20	8·97	1·64	(77·68, 86·71)

Figure 9   Minitab display giving basic description and 95% confidence interval for the mean tcpO$_2$ in forearm skin of a sample of 30 normal subjects. The first command gives the basic descriptive statistics, the second calculates by default the 95% confidence interval.

Comparative investigations

Many medical research investigations entail comparisons between subjects selected from various well defined subpopulations with the aim of detecting medically or scientifically significant differences between the overall distribution of certain variables in the different subpopulations. The simplest comparative investigation involves two subpopulations which may, for example, be a population of normal controls and a population of patients with a particular disease. Such an investigation would be carried out by randomly selecting roughly the same number of subjects from each subpopulation and making the appropriate measurement on each person. We will refer to this as the *two sample comparison*. A second, similar, type of investigation is known as the *paired comparison* investigation, in which the same measurement is made on each of several subjects twice—for example, before and after treatment—and so each subject acts as his or her own control for the purpose of assessing changes brought about by treatment. You must be careful to distinguish between the two types of comparative investigation because the appropriate statistical analyses are not interchangeable.

The analysis of the two sample comparison assumes that:

(i)   the measurements in each subpopulation are normally distributed;

(ii)   the difference between the subpopulations manifests itself only as a difference between the corresponding population means;

(iii)   the standard deviation is the same in both subpopulations.

In chapter 5 we shall describe alternative analyses to be used when these assumptions do not hold.

A confidence interval for the difference between the population means provides the answer to the question of whether the data show that the population means are different and it indicates how large the difference is likely to be.

The procedure is very similar to that used to determine a confidence interval in the single sample case. As an example, the data presented in fig 10 were obtained in an investigation that compared measurements of haemoglobin concentration in the blood of 80 healthy men and a similar group of 80 healthy women. The sample mean and standard deviation were 154·8 g/l and 24·9 g/l for the men, and the mean was 140·2 g/l and the standard deviation 28·1 g/l for the women. The difference between the sample means was 14·6 g/l and the standard error of this difference was 4·2 g/l. The 95% confidence interval for the difference between the population means stretches from 6·3 g/l to 22·9 g/l. This is interpreted as indicating that you can be 95% sure that average haemoglobin concentration in men can be expected to be between 6·3 g/l and 22·9 g/l higher than women. When there is only a small difference between population means—for example, in leucocyte counts, a similar investigation might produce the data

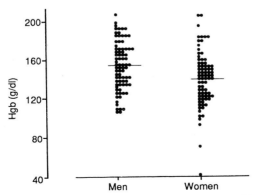

Figure 10   Haemoglobin concentration in men and women (80 subjects in each group).

27

illustrated in fig 11, with sample means of $6.97 \times 10^9/l$ and $7.04 \times 10^9/l$ and standard deviations of $1.05 \times 10^9/l$ and $0.95 \times 10^9/l$. A 95% confidence interval for the difference between the population mean for men and the population mean for women stretches from $-0.38 \times 10^9/l$ up to $0.24 \times 10^9/l$. In this case the supposition that there is no difference between the population means cannot be ruled out as zero falls inside the confidence interval.

The confidence interval is recommended as superior to *any* other method of statistical analysis in this situation because it gives a clear indication of the *size of the difference* between the population means, together with an equally clear indication of the *imprecision in our knowledge of the actual difference*. Thus there can be no doubt in the reader's mind as to whether a reported difference is medically important, because the probable size of the difference is quoted. Nor can there be much doubt about whether the sample sizes were large enough to detect worthwhile differences in an investigation which reports a "negative" finding—that is, a confidence interval which includes zero. For example, if a difference of 5 units would be medically significant but the confidence interval reported in a particular investigation stretched from -20 up to $+40$, its width indicates that variability is so great that a much larger investigation would be required to reduce the width of the interval to a level where you could be optimistic about detecting a difference of 5 units.

As an indication of how sample size affects the width of a

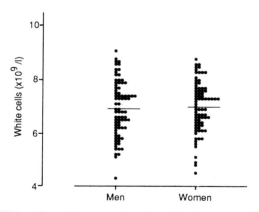

Figure 11   White cell counts in men and women (80 subjects in each group).

confidence interval, fig 12 shows the end points of 95% confidence intervals for investigations with the same means and standard deviations as in fig 10, and calculated from samples varying in size from 10 up to 500. The gain, in terms of decreased width, from using larger sample size is quite noticeable—up to 100 per group, but declines sharply thereafter.

The analysis of results arising from a paired comparison investigation can be summarised briefly, as no new ideas are involved. Recall that two measurements are made on each subject to estimate the difference between the population means before and after treatment. The appropriate method of analysis is to subtract the first measurement from the second for each subject and calculate a confidence interval for the mean of these differences. If the confidence interval does not straddle zero, this will indicate that treatment does affect the variable of interest.

Confidence intervals compared with significance tests

There is a strong association between the confidence interval approach and an alternative commonly used in the medical literature, based on the idea of a "significance test", in which the difference between the sample means is divided by the standard

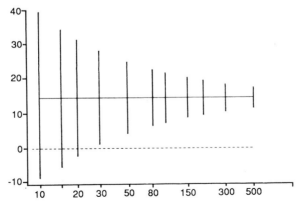

Figure 12   Effect of sample size on the width of a confidence interval. The bars represent confidence intervals for the difference in mean haemoglobin concentration using the means and standard deviations from the data of figure 10, but assuming sample sizes ranging from 10 up to 500 in each group.

error. The result is conventionally denoted by the symbol "*t*" and the method is known as the "*two sample t test*" (in the paired comparison, it is the mean of the differences divided by its standard error which is referred to as "*t*" and the corresponding test is the "*paired t test*").

The significance testing approach is based on the following argument: suppose the population means are equal, then we would expect the sample means to be roughly equal, apart from the inevitable difference resulting from sampling, and so their difference will be "close" to zero. The standard error of the difference is the appropriate scale factor for judging whether the observed difference is small enough for it to be regarded as evidence that the population means are equal. Thus "*t*" is the appropriate statistic for making the assessment. If "*t*" is large then this is taken as evidence against the supposition that the population means are equal. A "large" value is one which has a low probability of occurring when the population means are equal. This probability is called the p value in the medical literature and the significance level by statisticians.

The logic of the *t* test is as follows: if the p value associated with the result is small, say 0·01, then there are two possibilities:

(i) the population means *are equal* but the investigation has produced data which have only a 1 in 100 chance of occurring or;

(ii) the population means are not equal.

The conventional approach has been to regard an investigation as having produced evidence in favour of a genuine difference whenever the p value is less than 0·05, and then the result is reported as being "significant".

The shortcomings of the significance testing approach are well known to statisticians and have been pointed out on several occasions.[7][8] Firstly, the result of an investigation is being forced into a framework where all that matters is whether a result is or is not significant. This is surely not wise, as what really matters is whether an investigation has been able to detect a medically important difference between the population means and how large that difference is likely to be. Secondly, the significance test approach pretends that all situations can be neatly categorised as ones in which the population means are or are not exactly equal. In reality there is likely to be some difference between the population means, and so a very large investigation will stand a good chance of detecting the difference, no matter how small and medically unimportant it may be. The method can easily lead to the attitude that for example, a "significant $(p < 0.01)$" result should be interpreted as meaning that a difference which has a practical importance has been detected.

On the other hand, an investigation which results in a "not significant $(p < 0.05)$" difference risks being misinterpreted as providing conclusive evidence that a truly zero difference between the population means has been established. Nothing could be further from the truth. The correct interpretation is that any underlying difference is too small to have been detected by this particular investigation (the investigation may in fact have been too small to detect really worthwhile differences). Statistical analysis cannot be used to prove conclusively that there is absolutely no difference between a pair of population means.

By comparison the confidence interval approach is superior. As it gives a range of plausible values for the difference between the population means, the knowledgeable subject specialist is able to judge whether the difference being reported is of practical importance. In fact the confidence interval and the significance test are closely related. If the 95% confidence interval for the mean difference does not bracket zero, then the t test will produce a result which is significant at the 5% level and perhaps at an even lower level. Conversely, if the t test results in $p > 0.05$ then the 95% confidence interval will include zero, but the interval gives a more useful interpretation of the "not significant" result: the true difference may not be zero but could be any value within the interval.

As both the t test and the confidence interval approach are available in all good statistical packages it is advisable to combine the two. To illustrate this we compared the data of fig 10 using the "two sample" analysis from Statgraphics. The screen output is shown in fig 13; the major descriptive statistics for the two samples are shown in the top field. Note that both the standard deviations and the variances, which are merely the squares of the standard deviations, are displayed. Then the 95% confidence interval for the difference between the population means is given (the user can choose an alternative level such as 99%): the display next shows the results of two forms of the interval, the first being the one we have described above which assumes equal population standard deviations, the second is an alternative which is appropriate when the assumption is clearly invalid. The user may choose whichever

Two sample analysis results			
	HbM	HbF	Pooled
Sample Statistics: Number of Obs.	80	80	160
Average	154·817	140·238	147·528
Variance	622·298	789·773	706·035
Std. Deviation	24·9459	28·1029	26·5713
Median	154·9	141·9	147·7

Conf. Interval for Diff. in Means:	95 Percent		
(Equal Vars.)　　Sample 1 − Sample 2	6·28021 22·8798		158 D.F.
(Unequal Vars.)　Sample 1 − Sample 2	6·27931 22·8807		155·8 D.F.

Conf. Interval for Ratio of Variances:	95 Percent
Sample 1　　Sample 2	0·50532 1·22864

Hypothesis Test for H0: Diff = 0	Computed t statistic = 3·4703
vs Alt: NE	Sig. Level = 6·7024E–4
at Alpha = 0·05	so reject H0

Figure 13　Screen display produced by Statgraphics in response to a request for a two sample t test analysis of the haemoglobin data of figure 10.

is more appropriate, depending on the variances shown in the upper part of the panel. Thereafter the user has an opportunity for calculating a confidence interval for the ratio of the population variances at a probability level of his or her choice; this is a further guide to which of the alternative intervals to use. If the confidence interval for the ratio of the variances brackets the value one then the equal variance confidence interval is appropriate. The bottom section of the panel is written in computer statistics jargon, but we can interpret the computer output into plain English as follows: "the data provide evidence of a difference between mean haemoglobin concentrations in men and women. The difference between the sample means for two groups of 80 subjects was 14·6 g/l with a standard error of 4·2 g/l, this difference is significant at $p < 0.001$, and a 95% confidence interval for the difference between healthy men and women stretches from 6·3 g/l to 22·9 g/l".

This final display can be "dumped" to the printer for a permanent record at a single key stroke. With other simple manipulations, dot plots or box and whisker plots can be displayed and recorded permanently with a graph plotter. A bench-based laboratory scientist can thus obtain reliable comparisons between groups of experimental observations and to produce various forms of display to clarify the interpretation quickly on a microcomputer. Used properly this facility will extend the range and improve the efficiency of many types of laboratory work for a very small financial outlay.

4

Comparison of several groups: The analysis of variance

Comparison of several groups where distributions approximate to normal and where variances are similar

It is unusual for a biomedical research study to involve only comparison between two groups; more often the same observation is made on each subject in several groups with the aims of (i) detecting group differences and (ii) estimating their probable magnitudes. An example of this type of study is a comparison between haemoglobin concentrations in normal men (group A), normal women not receiving medication (group B), normal women taking the contraceptive pill (group C) and women with meno-metrorrhagia (group D) (fig 14).

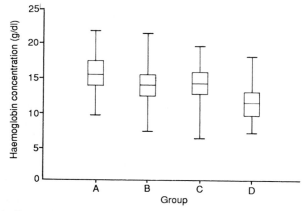

Figure 14   Box and whisker plots of the observed distribution of haemglobin concentration in random samples of 100 subjects from each of the following groups: (A) healthy men; (B) healthy women not receiving medication; (C) healthy women taking the contraceptive pill; (D) women with menometrorrhagia. All distributions seem to be symmetrical and variability is about the same in all groups.

A common, but inappropriate, method of analysis of such data entails the comparison of each pair of groups using the two sample t test to make each comparison. Thus group A is compared in turn with groups B, C, and D; group B is compared with groups C and D; and finally; group C is compared with D, resulting in a total of six t tests. This approach is basically flawed because it ignores the inherent associations in multiple comparisons and will inflate the chance of obtaining a misleading result. Remember that in the t test for comparison of two groups of data, the p value is the probability of obtaining a result at least as extreme as the observed difference between the sample means when there is no difference between the corresponding population means. Consequently, when applying a single t test at a p value of 0·05, the investigator has a 5% chance of being misled into concluding that there is evidence of a difference when the population means are equal and the observed extreme result is attributable entirely to the random variability of the responses. If two independent t tests are performed—for example, comparing A with B and C with D—in a situation where the corresponding population means are equal the probability that both will correctly indicate this is $0·95 \times 0·95$ or 0·9025 (90·25%), and so there is a 9·75% chance that at least one of the pair of tests will be misleading. If six comparisons were made (as in the haemoglobin study) and the corresponding population means were equal then the chance of a correct conclusion in all six tests is about $(0·95)^6$ or 0·735. In other words there is a greater than 1 in 4 chance that the result of at least one of the six tests will be misleading.

The probability of at least one misleading conclusion in a series of tests is known as the *error rate* of the series. The tendency for the error rate to rise rapidly as the number of groups increases means that the technique of pairwise comparisons cannot be recommended. Table 1 indicates the approximate error rate for comparison of several groups by pairwise t tests when it is proposed to report all results with p values of less than 0·05. Being more cautious and reporting only those results with p values less than 0·01 alleviates but does not entirely eliminate the problem.

The appropriate technique, *analysis of variance*,[3 4] not only takes full account of the multiple comparison nature of the problem but also uses the information in all samples to provide standard errors for the differences between pairs of population means (the pairwise t test method uses only information from the pair of samples being compared to determine the standard error of the difference).

TABLE 1

Overall error rates when several groups are compared by performing two sample t tests on all pairs of groups

No of groups	No of pairs	Overall error rate when the chosen significance level of each test is:	
		5%	1%
3	3	14%	3%
4	6	26%	6%
5	10	40%	10%
6	15	54%	14%
10	45	90%	36%

The method is available in both Statgraphics and Minitab. It is based on the following assumptions: (i) the variability within each group is about the same; (ii) observed values are more or less normally distributed within each population.

The basic principle is quite simple. If there are real differences between some of the population means, this will be reflected as differences between the corresponding sample means which will be significant if the study is large enough. In any investigation involving several groups the overall variability of the responses can be separated into two components: (i) variability between sample means, indicating possible differences between population means, and (ii) variability of responses within each group, indicating natural variability within each population. If the population means are equal then differences between the sample means will be entirely due to chance variations in the individual observations within each group so that the two types of variability (i) and (ii) ought to be comparable. If there are substantial differences between the population means, however, variability between sample means (i) ought to be considerably greater than variability within groups (ii).

The analysis of variance differentiates between these situations by making a direct comparison between (i) and (ii). For technical reasons the measure of spread used is not the standard deviation but its square, the variance. The method uses (a) the variance of the set of sample means and (b) an estimate of the natural variability based on the variances of the responses in each group, known as the "pooled" within groups variance, to calculate the variance ratio, or F-ratio, which is merely (a) divided by (b).

The evidence for or against differences between the population means of the various groups is assessed by determining the probability that a variance ratio at least as extreme as that actually observed could occur by chance if all the population means were equal—that is, the p value. A variance ratio which has a low p value is taken as evidence that real differences exist: by itself it does not indicate which sets are different from the remaining sets. The output from both packages is much the same and takes the form of a standard analysis of variance table (fig 15), which is part of the Statgraphics analysis of the data displayed in fig 14.

The analysis of variance is basically a significance testing procedure, so an F ratio which has a p value of less than 0.05 is conventionally taken as evidence of genuine differences between some of the population means. As usual the smaller p value the stronger is the evidence for differences. Thus in the haemoglobin example there is very strong evidence of differences between mean haemoglobin concentrations in some of the groups. Note that the analysis of variance, like all significance testing procedures, merely gives an indication of the strength of the evidence; it does not indicate which population means do differ or whether the differences are of practical, as distinct from statistical, significance.

Follow up analysis

To answer such questions it is essential to report the results of a "follow up" analysis. This can be done graphically by presenting appropriate confidence intervals for the population means. There

Analysis of variance					
Source of variation	Sum of squares	d.f.	Mean square	F-ratio	Sig. level
Between groups	865·4021	3	288·4674	43·8941	0·0000
Within groups	2602·4706	396	6·5719		
Total (corrected)	3467·8727	399			

Figure 15   The analysis of variance table produced by Statgraphics for the data summarised in figure 14. F-ratio is highly significant (the value 0·0000 displayed under "Sig. level" means that the p value is less than 0·00005), indicating that the data provide extremely strong evidence of differences between the population means of some groups. It is not possible to tell from this table which groups differ.

are various methods of doing this. Minitab displays individual 95% confidence intervals for the means using essentially the same method as that used for a two sample investigation, but with the important proviso that the standard error for the difference between any pair of means is derived from information on variability obtained from *all* samples and not merely from the two samples being compared. The analysis of variance and follow up produced by Minitab are displayed in fig 16. This shows that (i) healthy men have a higher mean haemoglobin concentration than women; (ii) women taking the contraceptive pill have a mean haemoglobin concentration which cannot be distinguished from that of healthy women not receiving medication, and (iii) women with menometrorrhagia have a mean haemoglobin concentration that is significantly lower than that of healthy women.

Analysis of variance		haemoglobin		
Source	DF	SS	MS	F
Groups	3	865·40	288·47	43·89
Error	396	2602·47	6·57	
Total	399	3467·87		
Group	N	Mean	STDEV	
A	100	15·659	2·572	
B	100	13·943	2·612	
C	100	14·156	2·559	
D	100	11·552	2·511	

Pooled STDEV= 2·564

Individual 95 PCT CI's for mean based on pooled STDEV

Figure 16   The analysis of variance table provided by Minitab also includes a graphical follow up analysis. 95% confidence intervals for the population means of the four groups are interpreted in the usual way: intervals which do not overlap indicate a difference between the corresponding population means.

The Statgraphics package produces a similar follow up analysis on request but tabulates the confidence limits rather than displaying them graphically. An extra follow up feature of Statgraphics is its ability to indicate those sample means for which there is no evidence of a difference between the corresponding population means (fig 17). In the section of the table headed "homogeneous groups" asterisks in the same column alongside the means for groups B and C indicate that they do not differ significantly. The technique used for for these calculations is known as a *multiple comparisons procedure*[9] and several alternative methods are available within Statgraphics, differing mainly in the details of calculations involved in producing the final result. Which one is used is largely immaterial because all will give very similar results. What is important is that some form of follow up analysis should always be performed after obtaining a significant F-ratio in the initial analysis of variance.

Diagnostic plots

The analysis of variance is based on assumptions of homogeneity of spread of responses in the various groups and normality of the distribution of responses. Failure of the responses to conform to these assumptions, either directly or via the presence of outliers, may result in the analysis of variance being misleading. The assumptions may be checked by examining the *residuals*, which are the deviations of the responses from the corresponding group means. The most useful plots are (i) a plot of residuals against the group means and (ii) a normal plot of the residuals (chapter 2). Residuals which are particularly large may indicate outliers. Repeating the analysis with suspect observations omitted will

Multiple range analysis for haemoglobin by group			
Method: Group	95 Percent Count	Scheffe Average	Homogeneous Groups
A	100	15·659	
C	100	14·156	*
B	100	13·943	*
D	100	11·552	

Figure 17   Statgraphics provides an alternative follow up analysis based on multiple comparison methods.

39

indicate whether they play a large part in determining the conclusions.

The plot of residuals against the group means (an additional option in Statgraphics) is very similar to the plot of the raw data which should be the starting point of the analysis of variance, except that each group of residuals is centred on zero and so visual comparison is easier. The danger sign to look out for is either one group of residuals with a much greater spread than the rest, or a tendency for the spread to vary appreciably and systematically over the groups. If either pattern appears then the assumption of uniform spread is not tenable and some corrective action such as a transformation of the data may be needed. The normal plot of the residuals should be nearly a straight line if the data conform to the normality assumption, but curvature can indicate non-normality, inhomogeneity of spread, or the presence of outliers: it is therefore wise to look at both plots. Both packages calculate residuals and fitted values on demand and so the two diagnostic plots can easily be obtained.

The broader problem of multiple testing

In many investigations various observations are made on subjects belonging to different categories and these may then be analysed in a number of ways to suggest fruitful areas for concentration of further research effort. With a large and complex data set there are likely to be several hundred ways in which various combinations of variables may be analysed. The problem of overall error rates and multiple comparisons is obviously important here, for if every result with a p value of 0·05 or less is reported as corresponding to a genuine difference, then 1 in 20 (5%) of the reported results may be misleading in the sense of indicating a difference where one does not exist. Partly, the problem arises from the use of a significance test as an exploratory tool in sifting through a large body of data: a function for which it is not ideally suited. The proportion of spuriously significant results among a large group of tests may be reduced by resisting the temptation to report *every* result with a p value of less than 0·05, reporting instead only those results with p values of less than 0·01 or some similar figure: using 0·05 divided by the square root of the number of tests performed gives a p value which is a reasonable compromise between spurious significance and being over-stringent. Alternatively, you may adopt the viewpoint that the statistical tests performed in an exploratory situation are merely being used to generate interesting hypotheses which must be confirmed in a further investigation of at least the same size as that from which they were derived.

Replicates and repeated measures

REPLICATES

Whenever a method of measurement is indirect and is the result of a complex process of sample preparation it is customary for the investigator to replicate each sample. For instance, in measuring uptake of ^{3}H-TdR as an indicator of DNA synthesis it is common practice to make triplicate preparations from each sample at the same time and to measure each one. This is a recognition of the fact that the process of sample preparation and the measurement of the amount of radioactive tracer introduces quite a substantial amount of experimental variability which is extremely difficult to control. When this is so the mean of the values from the three replicates is likely to be closer to the underlying absolute value than any one of the values. The standard deviation of the values, which may be referred to as the replicates standard deviation, gives an indication of the variability resulting from the process of sample preparation and measurement. If the replication is performed for each subject then the replicates standard deviation for each subject can be combined to provide a more precise measurement of experimental variability.

Information about the magnitude of the experimental variability is useful in planning further investigations but it is often incidental to the main aim of a study which is likely to be the comparison of different groups of subjects. It is therefore imperative to make a clear distinction between variability between subjects, which is used to obtain an estimate of population variability, and variability between replicates from which an estimate of experimental variability can be obtained. It is the population variability not the experimental variability which is relevant to assessing whether groups differ. When equal replication for all subjects is possible then the simplest way of comparing groups is to perform an analysis of variance of the means of the replicates. When the amount of replication is not the same for each subject then a more complex analysis is required and you would be wise to consult a statistician.

REPEATED MEASURES

One form of repeated measures study involves a series of measurements made over a period of time on each one of a number of subjects in one or more groups. The type of question which the investigation is set up to answer is concerned with whether the way in which subject response changes with time differs from one group to another and, if this is so, what is it that characterises the differences. The measurements in each series, although made on the same subject, are in no sense replicates as you expect any differences between measurements made at different times to be due to changes in the absolute level of the quantity being measured and not solely attributable to experimental error as is the case with replicates.

Because a series of measurements is made on each subject, the data arising from such a study do not conform to the basic assumptions of most univariate methods of analysis which assume that each value is independent of the rest. This cannot be the case here, for a subject who starts with an initially high value is likely to continue to have high values and so the measurements on one subject will be correlated. In most cases the appropriate techniques are those of *multivariate analysis*.

Repeated measures studies are inherently more difficult to analyse and the results of the analysis are more difficult to comprehend precisely because you are trying to understand and characterise a series of correlated measurements. It is often the case that a repeated measures study is incorrectly analysed by ignoring the fact that the measurements on a single subject are related and then using a univariate analysis of variance of the type described in this chapter. This is not recommended because it oversimplifies the true situation to such an extent that the results of the analysis are likely to be quite misleading. The correct analysis requires a familiarity with the techniques of multivariate analysis of variance and so is outside the scope of this book. The advice of your local statistical guru should be sought before embarking on a repeated measures type of study.

5

Analysis of continuous data that are not normally distributed: Distribution free methods

The various statistical techniques described in the previous chapters are based on assumptions concerning the distribution of responses. In particular, outliers or extreme non-normality may seriously influence the results of any analysis which relies on the normality assumption. Normal plots of the raw data in each sample or of the residuals can be used to assess how well the data conform, provided the sample sizes are sufficiently large (chapter 2). This method is insensitive with small samples, however, as only the most extreme forms of non-normality will be detected. Fortunately, both the methods based on the t test and the analysis of variance are pretty robust as far as moderate departures from normality are concerned.

Some types of non-normality may be corrected by an appropriate transformation such as the logarithmic or the square root transformation. If a transformation to correct non-normality cannot be found, then an alternative approach is available. A significance test and the appropriate confidence interval may be determined by using distribution free (or non-parametric) methods.[10][11] These methods do not assume that the population distributions are "normal", but assume instead that the distribution shape is about the same in each population being compared.

We recommend the following procedure for deciding whether to use a distribution free procedure. First, see whether a transformation will achieve near normality. Make the transformation, and plot the transformed data looking at both the normal probability plot and the box and whisker plot. If these plots show no serious departures from normality, in other words the points on the normal plot lie more or less on a straight line and the box and whisker plot is symmetrical, then the transformation has achieved its purpose. It is therefore safe to analyse the *transformed data* by methods which are based on the assumption that the underlying distribution is normal. When reporting the results of the analysis you will have to back-transform any descriptive statistics or confidence intervals that are used so as to make them refer to the original data. If there does not seem to be a transformation which works then the data should be analysed by the appropriate distribution free method.

There is a widespread belief that distribution free methods can be applied to any data because they make no assumptions whatsoever about the underlying data distribution but this is not correct. The true state of affairs is that these methods do make some assumptions such as symmetry or that the shapes of the underlying distributions are the same. These assumptions are not so restrictive as the normality assumption, but they are implicit in the methods and must be more or less valid for the methods to be applied safely.

Distribution free equivalent of the *t* test

The median is a more appropriate indicator of location than the mean for appreciably asymmetrical non-normal distributions, so the two sample distribution free significance test assesses the evidence for a difference between the population medians: the distribution free confidence interval represents a range of plausible values for this difference.

The relevant method for *two sample comparisons* is known as the *Mann-Whitney procedure*. It is based on the principle of replacing the actual data values by their ranks. First, the two samples are combined and sorted into ascending order. Then the observations are ranked giving rank 1 to the smallest, rank 2 to the next smallest, and so on. If two or more observations are equal then the average of the ranks which would be assigned is allocated to each one.

The test statistic used to assess evidence for a difference between the population medians is the sum of the ranks in the first sample and is often designated by the letter W. The value of W reflects the relative position of the two sets of sample values. If the values in the first sample tend to be higher than those in the second sample then the larger ranks will occur predominantly in the first sample and W will be large. Obviously W will be small if the values in the first sample tend to be smaller than those in the second sample. For example, box plots of the survival times of two groups of patients with breast cancer are shown in fig 18. Group A comprises patients with 40% or more of malignant cells in sections of neoplastic tissue and group B patients with less than 40% of malignant cells. The plots suggest that survival may be related to percentage of malignant cells in the sense that survival seems to be somewhat longer in group B. The output from Minitab, consisting of a basic description of the data, the Mann-Whitney test, and a confidence interval for the difference between the population medians is displayed in fig 19. Although the median of group B is larger than that of group A, the probability of obtaining a difference in medians at least as large as this when the population medians are equal is 0·25 and consequently the difference is not significant. The conclusion is clear: the data fail to provide statistically acceptable evidence of a difference between population median survival times for the two groups.

The distribution free confidence interval for the difference between the population medians is based on the calculation of all the differences between the survival times for the first group and those for the second group. As this procedure is not widely known

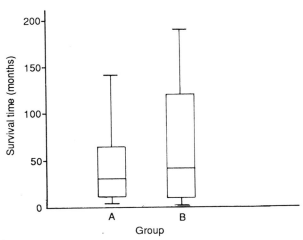

Figure 18   Box and whisker plots of the survivals of patients with breast cancer in a retrospective study of the use of morphometric features as predictors of survival. The distributions are extremely asymmetrical and so median survival is more informative than mean survival. This degree of asymmetry rules out the use of methods based on the normal distribution.

an example of how the calculations are performed is given in the Appendix. The observed medians for the two groups are 30 months and 41 months, and you might therefore think that the best estimate of the difference between the medians of the underlying populations was merely the difference between the group medians. Unfortunately, this is not the case; the best estimate is in fact the median of all the pairwise differences between survival times. A little experimentation with some small sets of data will soon convince the reader that the difference between the medians of two groups is not the same as the median of the differences between pairs of values with one value from each group. This can be seen in fig 19, where the point estimate for the difference between the population medians based on the data for the two groups is − 12 months, a negative value because all the evidence seems to indicate that the population corresponding to group B has a higher median. Note, however, that the confidence interval for the difference

```
MTB > DESCRIBE 'GROUP-A' 'GROUP-B'

          N   MEAN   MEDIAN  STDEV  MIN    MAX     Q1     Q3
GROUP-A   30  39·03  30·00   35·81  3·00   142·00  10·75  64·75
GROUP-B   32  64·70  41·00   59·40  0·00   191·00  9·20   121·20

MTB > MANNWHITNEY 'GROUP-A' 'GROUP-B'

Mann-Whitney Confidence Interval and Test

GROUP-A  N = 30  MEDIAN = 30·000
GROUP-B  N = 32  MEDIAN = 41·000
POINT ESTIMATE FOR ETA1–ETA2 IS  − 11·9986
95·1 PCT C.I. FOR ETA1–ETA2 IS (− 50, 5)
W = 862·0
TEST OF ETA1 = ETA2 VS. ETA1 N.E. ETA2 IS SIGNIFICANT AT
0·2452

CANNOT REJECT AT ALPHA = 0·05
```

Figure 19   Minitab display of basic descriptive statistics and the distribution free Mann-Whitney analysis of the data summarised in figure 18. "ETA1" and "ETA2" are Minitab jargon for the population medians for the two groups. The 95% confidence interval for the true difference between the population medians includes zero, indicating that there is insufficient evidence to claim a real difference between median survival time. This is confirmed by the p value (0·2452) associated with W. The phrase "cannot reject at alpha = 0·05" indicates that a significance test at the conventional level of 5% fails to reject the hypothesis that the population medians are equal.

between the population medians is -50 months up to 5 months. This can be interpreted as meaning that the data are somewhat equivocal, and can do no more than indicate that, firstly, there is a possibility that the population medians could be equal, as zero months falls within the interval, and secondly, that the population median for group B could be up to 50 months more than that of group A or could be up to 5 months less. The fact that no difference between population medians is not precluded by the confidence interval calculation is in line with the conclusion derived from the Mann-Whitney significance test. Statgraphics is not so useful in this situation; it is capable of performing the Mann-Whitney test, but does not provide the corresponding confidence interval.

A similar distribution free technique for the *paired sample comparison* is known as the *Wilcoxon technique*. Recall that a typical paired comparison investigation involves two measurements made on each subject, and the appropriate analysis involves examining the differences between the paired observations.

First, the observed differences are ordered, ignoring their signs. Ranks are then assigned in the usual way and each rank is then given the same sign as the corresponding difference. The test statistic for assessing evidence that the median of the population distribution of differences is non-zero is the sum of the signed ranks. A value close to zero indicates no real difference between the pairs of measurements, whereas a large value (positive or negative) may be evidence of genuine differences. If the p value associated with the signed rank statistic is less than 0·05 then this is taken as evidence of genuine differences between the first and second response. There is a corresponding method of calculating a confidence interval for the population median difference between the paired responses. Both Minitab and Statgraphics perform the Wilcoxon signed rank test, but only Minitab provides the confidence interval. The Appendix describes the method for calculation of the confidence interval for the benefit of Statgraphics users.

As the distribution free techniques do not take account of the actual data values, but merely their relative positions, they are much more resistant to the effects of outliers than the corresponding techniques based on the t statistic. They thus provide at least a partial remedy to the thorny problem of whether to omit apparent outliers from an analysis.

There is a common misconception that distribution free

47

methods make no assumptions whatsoever about the data to which they may be applied and so there is a tendency to apply them in all situations, even when they are inappropriate. It is commonly stated that almost all biomedical data are non-normally distributed and so methods which have a built-in assumption of normality are of no value. This exaggerates the true situation and also ignores the fact that when data conform reasonably well with the assumption of normality, the t based techniques are not seriously misleading and are in fact slightly more *powerful*, in the sense of being able to detect smaller differences. Moreover, when they are appropriate, t based confidence intervals will be narrower than distribution free intervals. Thus our strong recommendation is to use the appropriate technique: if there is no evidence that the data are seriously out of line with the usual assumptions use the t based methods and reserve distribution free techniques for remedial cases.

Distribution free analysis of variance

As with the two sample situation, there is a distribution free technique which may be used in the event of serious non-conformity with the normality assumption, either through asymmetry or outliers which cannot be corrected. The method is the *Kruskal-Wallis test* and like the Mann-Whitney test it is based on ranks. The data from all groups are combined and ranked, then the mean rank is calculated for each group. The test statistic measures how far apart these mean ranks are and statistical theory indicates how large the Kruskal-Wallis statistic is likely to be when there are no real differences between the corresponding population medians. To illustrate the technique the Kruskal-Wallis method is applied to the haemoglobin data of fig 14, even though these data are normally distributed, and the corresponding output from Statgraphics is displayed in fig 20. The mean ranks for the four groups are somewhat different, and the extremely small p value of the Kruskal-Wallis statistic indicates that there are differences among some of the groups. Unfortunately, the utility of the Kruskal-Wallis method is somewhat reduced because neither package provides a follow up analysis and there is no easy way of obtaining distribution free confidence intervals for the group medians. One way round this is to apply either the signed rank method (see appendix) to produce individual confidence intervals for each population median, or to use the Mann-Whitney based method to

Kruskal-Wallis analysis of haemoglobin by group		
Group	Sample Size	Average Rank
A	100	270·9000
B	100	204·8000
C	100	216·3000
D	100	109·9000
Test statistic = 100·5000	Significance level = 3·702E–6	

Figure 20   Statgraphics display for the Kruskal-Wallis analysis of the data summarised in figure 14. The average ranks for the four groups differ appreciably. The p value of the Kruskal-Wallis statistic T is extremely small so the analysis indicates extremely strong evidence of differences between groups which agrees with the analysis of variance and follow up analyses displayed in figures 15–71.

obtain confidence intervals for differences between all pairs of group medians.

The former is marginally simpler to apply than the latter, but either will only be useful when the sample sizes are reasonably large (more than 10 per group as a rough guide), and even in this case the procedure will tend to be rather conservative because there is nothing analogous to the residual mean square for gaining extra precision by using information from all samples in determining the standard error as in the analysis of variance. In the event of there being serious doubts about whether the standard method is applicable then the best advice is to consult your friendly, local statistical guru.

Appendix

The Mann-Whitney confidence interval for the difference between two medians

A simple example will make the method clear. Suppose two samples of responses are (in ascending order),

group A 56, 57, 58, 61, 62, 63, 66, 69 – median 61·5
group B 42, 48, 50, 51, 53, 54, 59   – median 51·0

All possible arithmetical differences between responses in group A and group B are calculated. This is most easily done by constructing a table bordered by the ordered responses with the minimum values in the "north-west" corner, entering the corresponding differences in the body of the table as shown on page 51.

The 95% confidence interval is formed by eliminating the m smallest and m largest values from this table, where the value of m is determined by consulting a table of percentage points of the Mann-Whitney distribution.[12] In this example the 10 smallest and 10 largest values must be eliminated. These values are marked with asterisks in the table. The smallest of the remaining values is 4 and the largest is 16, so the 95% confidence interval for the difference between group medians stretches from 4 to 16.

The calculations are rather tedious done by hand, but they can be shortened by noting that with the above type of tabulation the largest and smallest differences will always appear in the north-east and south-west corners of the table and so it is not necessary to calculate all differences. With a little ingenuity the calculations can be done with a spreadsheet program. Readers with some knowledge of BASIC programming should be able to construct a small program to perform the calculations.

Wilcoxon signed rank based interval

Suppose the differences between paired responses in each of 8 subjects were:

-4, 1, 5, 7, 9, 10, 12, 16.

The confidence interval for the median difference is obtained in a somewhat similar manner to the Mann-Whitney interval. A table is constructed, bordered by the ordered differences with the minimum value in the north-west corner, and the entries in the table are the averages of the corresponding row and column values, as shown below—for example, the entry in row 3, column 5 is $(5+9)/2 = 7$. It is necessary only to complete the upper half of the table to obtain all the necessary values because the lower half is merely a repetition of the upper portion. The 95% confidence level is obtained by eliminating the m smallest and m largest averages: the value of m is obtained from a table of the percentage points of the Wilcoxon signed ranks distribution,[12] the interval stretches from the smallest to the largest of the remaining averages. In this case the appropriate value of m is 3 and so the 95% confidence interval stretches from 1 up to 12·5.

		Group B						
		42	48	50	51	53	54	59
	56	14	8	6	5	3*	3*	−3*
	57	15	9	7	6	4*	3*	−2*
Group	58	16	10	8	7	5	4*	−1*
A	61	19*	13	11	10	8	7	2*
	62	20*	14	12	11	9	8	3*
	63	21*	15	13	12	10	9	4
	66	24*	18*	16	15	13	12	7
	69	27*	21*	19*	18*	16*	15	10

	−4	1	5	7	9	10	12	16
−4	−4·0*	−1·5*	0·5*	1·5	2·5	3·0	4·0	6·0
1		1·0	3·0	4·0	5·0	5·5	6·5	8·5
5			5·0	6·0	7·0	7·5	8·5	10·5
7				7·0	8·0	8·5	9·5	11·5
9					9·0	9·5	10·5	12·5
10						10·0	1·0	13·0*
12							12·0	14·0*
16								16.0*

6

Are variables related? Correlation and regression

Correlation

An important aspect of the statistical analysis of large quantities of measured data is the identification of patterns within the data. In this chapter elementary techniques for describing relations between pairs of continuous variables will be examined. A typical investigation will result in data which consist of measurements of several different variables on a sample of subjects. If certain variables can be shown to be related, in the sense that knowledge of the value of one variable enables an approximate value to be predicted for another, then (a) the description of the data can be simplified and (b) the fact that there is a relation may lead to interesting hypotheses about the mechanisms which cause the variables to be related.

Preliminary scatter plots should always be used to assess visually whether a pair of variables seem to be related and to indicate roughly the strength of that relation. The points on a particular plot may seem to be randomly scattered (fig 21A), clustered about a straight line (fig 21B), or a curve (fig 21C). Very roughly, a relation is strong if the scatter plot defines the line or curve more or less exactly with very little scatter, but is weaker if the points are more widely scattered.

The statistical measure of relation (or association) most commonly used in the biomedical literature is the *product-moment correlation coefficient*, usually abbreviated to the *correlation coefficient* and commonly denoted by the symbol "r". This is an objective measure of the strength of a linear relation between two variables and is a dimensionless number—that is, it is not affected by a change of units of measurement—which always takes a value in the range -1 to $+1$. The extremes of this range correspond to a

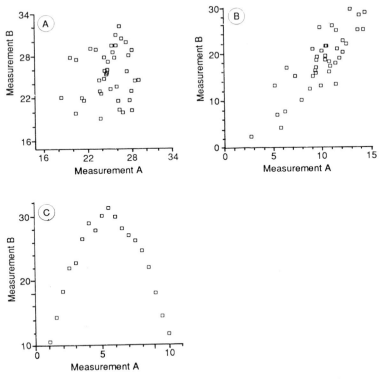

Figure 21 Scatter plots of hypothetical data illustrating (A) no relation between measurements A and B (r = 0·129; p > 0·10; (B) a linear relation between measurements A and B (r = 0·84; p < 0·001); (C) a curved relation between measurements A and B (r = 0·021; p > 0·1).

perfect linear relation between the variables, a situation which will not occur in practice. It is important to realise that this type of analysis is appropriate only in situations where the relation is linear (fig 21B) and so it would not be correct to use it in situations similar to that illustrated by fig 21C where the correlation coefficient is close to zero but there is a strong non-linear relation between the measurements. With this proviso, a correlation close to zero, corresponding to a scatter plot similar to that depicted in fig 21A will indicate that there is no relation between the corresponding variables.

The Statgraphics correlation analysis procedure may be used to generate a table of correlations between all pairs of variables in a list entered by the user; each correlation coefficient is displayed with the corresponding sample size and p value. A similar procedure is provided in Minitab but as p values are not given a table of percentage points of the correlation coefficient must be consulted.[12] The p value relates to the test of the hypothesis of no linear relation between the variables; consequently, a correlation coefficient which has a low p value indicates the existence of a linear relation. One of the difficulties of intepreting a significant correlation is that it is difficult to form an impression of how much clustering a correlation of, say, 0·70 represents. It cannot be interpreted as about 70% of what you would expect when there is a perfect linear relation; indeed it is difficult to understand what this might mean. One solution is to look at the square of the correlation coefficient, which represents the proportion of the variability in the measured values of one parameter, which is explained by its linear relation with the other parameter. Thus a significant correlation coefficient of 0·7 would indicate that about 50% of the variability in one parameter is explained by its linear relation with the other. Whether this is good or poor will depend on the question you are trying to answer by calculating the correlation coefficient. As we shall see later there are circumstances in which a correlation coefficient of 0·965, although highly impressive, completely fails to provide the answer to the question being posed. Whether a particular result is significant depends on the sample size: a correlation of 0·2 is significant at the 5% level if the sample size exceeds 100, yet on squaring this value we see that the supposed linear relation explains only about 4% of the variability in either parameter, or to put it more forcefully, 96% of the variability is not explained. This emphasises once more that more attention should be paid to the practical (clinical or biological) meaning of a result than to significance in this type of analysis.

The p value of the significance test is calculated on the assumption that the underlying population distribution of each variable is a normal distribution. The test is reasonably robust to departures from normality,[13 14] but it is not robust to the presence of outliers; a single badly placed point in conjunction with an otherwise random cloud of points can produce a highly significant correlation. This situation is illustrated in fig 22A; the correlation coefficient for all the data is 0·65, which is highly significant. If the outlying point is omitted the value falls to 0·07, which is not significant. In this

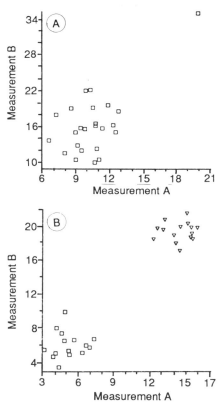

Figure 22   Scatter plots illustrating situations where the correlation coefficient is misleading: (A) the presence of a single outlier seriously influences the value of the correlation coefficient, with the outlier r = 0·65, omitting the outlier r = 0·007; (B) the data for men (squares) and women (triangles) fall into two separate groups. The correlation coefficient for all the data is 0·955, spuriously indicating a relation between measurements A and B. For men alone, r = 0·075 and for women alone r = 0·062, indicating that when sex is taken into account the measurements are not related.

situation it would be most unwise to take the larger correlation as "evidence" of an association between the variables.

When data refer to two or more groups with different character-istics—for example, men and women—then the correlation coeffi-cient may incorrectly indicate a significant linear relation between variables when the scatter plot (fig 22B) shows the presence of two or more separate groups within each of which the variables are not related. The spuriously significant correlation arises because the centres of the clouds of points lie on a straight line.

Rank correlation

If a scatter plot indicates a curved relation then the product-moment correlation coefficient will be inappropriate. Moderate curvature may often be removed by log-transforming one or both variables. An alternative is the *rank correlation coefficient* which may be used when the scatter plot indicates a "monotonic" curve. Monotonic means either that as the x variable increases so does the y variable, or that as the x variable increases the y variable decreases. Obviously a straight line is a special case of a monotonic "curve". The underlying curve indicated by the points in fig 2C is not monotonic as y first increases and then decreases as x increases. The rank correlation is the ordinary product-moment correlation calculated using the ranks of the two sets of observations when they are separately sorted into ascending order instead of the original data. The corresponding significance test does not require normality of the underlying distributions and also provides considerable protection against the malign influence of outliers. For example, the rank correlation coefficient for the data of fig 22A is 0·045, which is not significant; the influence of the outlying point has been attenuated.

The interpretation of a significant rank correlation is that there is a monotonic relation between the variables. There are problems of interpretation of the rank correlation coefficient similar to those encountered with the product-moment correlation coefficient; a rank correlation of 0·2 will be significant in samples of size 100 but this may not represent a practically important relation. Although not strictly valid, the interpretation of the square of the rank correlation as being an indication of the variability explained by the monotonic relation should be borne in mind.

Multiple comparisons

Correlation coefficients are generally overused and they should be avoided for anything other than exploration of the data because they are difficult to interpret correctly, and significant correlations may occur when the relation between the variables is so weak as to be practically useless.

Examination of a large number of variables by routine calculation of the correlations between all possible pairs, with all those which are significant at the 5% level being reported, should be avoided because this procedure is likely to be extremely misleading. For example, in a study in which 30 variables are measured on each of 200 subjects there are 435 correlations between pairs of variables ($30 \times 29/2$). Of these, you would expect 22 (5% of 435) to be spuriously significant at the 5% level and an additional 4 or 5 to be spuriously significant at the 1% level. Spuriously significant means falsely indicating an association when the corresponding pair of variables are not related. Both Minitab and Statgraphics can produce tables of correlations between all possible pairs of variables, together with the corresponding p values in the case of Statgraphics. In view of the serious problems arising from the multiple comparisons inherent in this procedure extreme care is needed in interpreting the results. The wise course is to ignore all those correlation coefficients which do not have very small p values 0·001 or less); otherwise, one is likely to report and then go on to discuss and perhaps even provide speculative explanations for a large number of spuriously significant correlations.

Linear regression analysis

Linear regression analysis is a powerful and widely applicable technique for fitting straight lines or certain types of curves to data and assessing how well the fitted model describes the data. The method is used to fit a linear relation between two variables, one of which is known as the *response variable*, or y variable, the other being referred to as the *explanatory variable*, or x variable.

The decision as to which variable is the response and which is explanatory depends on the context of the investigation. Sometimes it is quite obvious which is which. For example, in looking at changes over time (fig 23), where acinar volume is plotted against age, it is clear that age must be the explanatory variable. In an investigation of the response of PHA stimulated lymphocytes to different concentrations of a particular steroidal drug, concentration must be the explanatory variable. In other situations the decision may not be so clear cut, the relation between height and weight in a group of subjects of the same age and sex being a classic example. Depending on the purpose of the investigation there could be two objectives; given a subject's height you might want to

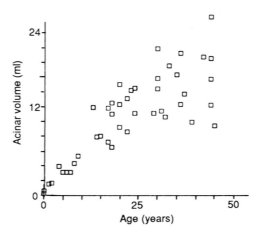

Figure 23 Scatter plot of acinar volume against age. There is some suggestion of curvature and an obvious indication that variability increases with age.

say something about their likely weight, or given a subject's weight you might want to predict their likely height. In the first situation it is sensible to take height as the explanatory variable, but in the second, height should be taken as the response variable.

In using simple linear regression analysis the aim is to explain at least part of the variability in the response variable values by means of the model:

$$\begin{bmatrix} \text{value of} \\ \text{response} \\ \text{variable} \end{bmatrix} = \text{intercept} + \text{slope} \times \begin{bmatrix} \text{value of} \\ \text{explanatory} \\ \text{variable} \end{bmatrix} + \begin{bmatrix} \text{unexplained} \\ \text{residual} \\ \text{amount} \end{bmatrix}$$

The various parts of this model are illustrated in fig 24. The intercept and slope are often referred to as the parameters of the line. It must be emphasised that this is only the simplest of the regression models available for relating values of a response variable to values of explanatory variables; polynomial regression may be used to fit curved relations and multiple regression may be used to find a small set of explanatory variables which together provide a good prediction of a response.

The model assumes that the values of the explanatory variable are known exactly; examples of variables for which this condition is likely to be true are age, volume of an organ or tumour determined after excision, body weight and basically all measure-

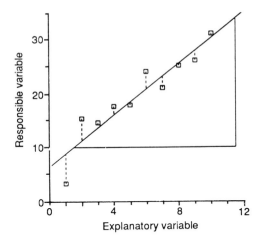

Figure 24   Diagram illustrating the components of the linear regression model. The slope of the fitted line is the ratio of two sides of the triangle (vertical/horizontal), the intercept is the value of the response predicted by the fitted line when the value of the explanatory variable is zero, the broken lines joining the data points to the fitted line indicate the residuals.

ments of quantities which show long term stability made directly with some instrument that has extremely small instrumental error. The component labelled "unexplained residual" in the model may be due to instrumental error in the measurement of the response variable, or it may represent biological variability between subjects who happen to have the same value for the explanatory variable, or it may be a combination of both.

As an example, we shall consider an investigation of the relation between total volume of the acinar units in the normal thyroid gland and age. Ideally, such a study should be conducted by measuring the response variable for equal numbers of subjects at each chosen age point as both the average level and the variability of the response variable may be related to age. The data displayed in fig 23 are therefore less than ideal because early ages are underrepresented but they will serve to illustrate the essentials of the analysis. Visual inspection shows that there is a clear relation between acinar volume and age, but variability also seems to be related to age. The output of the Statgraphics simple linear regression module for these data is shown in fig 25. Interpretation of the top part of the table is straightforward. The fitted linear relation is:

Regression Analysis – Linear Model: $Y = a + bX$				
Dependent variable: avol			Independent variable: age	
Parameter	Estimate	Standard error	T Value	Prob. level
Intercept	2·89593	0·993577	2·94428	5·2562E–3
Slope	0·341179	0·0369029	9·24533	1·10669E–11
Analysis of Variance				
Source	Sum of Squares	Df	Mean Square	F-Ratio	Prob. Level
Model	937·25108	1	937·25108	85·47606	·00000
Error	460·53296	42	10·96507		

Total
(Corr.)   1397·7840   43
Correlation Coefficient = 0·818857   R-squared = 67·05 percent
Stnd. Error of Est. = 3·31135

Figure 25   Statgraphics display of the results of fitting a straight line to the data of figure 23.

$$\text{acinar volume} = 2{\cdot}90 + 0{\cdot}34 \times \text{age}$$

while the standard errors indicate the precision of the corresponding parameters and provide the information needed for tests of the hypotheses that the population intercept and slope are zero. Under the heading "T-value" are the estimates divided by their standard errors, the values under "Prob. level" indicate the probability of obtaining t values as extreme as those observed in a situation where the corresponding population parameter is zero. As in most situations where the scatter plot indicates an association the investigator will expect the slope to be non-zero, this t test is not very informative unless zero turns out to be a plausible value for the slope, in which case the conclusion would be that the data contain no evidence of a linear relation between the variables. Confidence intervals are usually more informative and take the form

$$\begin{bmatrix} \text{parameter} \\ \text{estate} \end{bmatrix} \pm \begin{bmatrix} \text{standard} \\ \text{error} \end{bmatrix} \times \begin{bmatrix} \text{percentage point of} \\ \text{the } t \text{ distribution} \end{bmatrix}$$

The 95% confidence interval for the slope is obtained by looking up the 5% point of the t distribution in a set of statistical tables; the number of degrees of freedom required is shown in the Statgraphics output in the row labelled "error" under the "Df" column (42 in this case). In this example the percentage point value is 2·02 and so the 95% confidence interval for the slope parameter stretches from 0·27 to 0·42.

The analysis of variance table divides the total variability in the response values, which is the value under "Sum of Squares" in the row labelled "Total" into components attributable to the model and the unexplained residual. The "mean squares" are the corresponding sums of squares divided by their degrees of freedom and the "F-ratio" is the model mean square divided by the error mean square. In this example the F-ratio is large and the value under "prob. level" indicates that the chance of getting so large an F-ratio is very small if there is no relation between acinar volume and age. Accordingly, we may conclude that the data provide extremely strong evidence of a relation. The correlation coefficient needs no explanation, more informative is the value labelled "R-squared" which is the square of the correlation coefficient and indicates that 67% of the variability in acinar volume can be explained by the linear relation with age.

A further useful graphical display generated on request by Statgraphics is shown in fig 26. As the fitted line is estimated from a sample of 44 subjects there will be some uncertainty about the true average acinar volume at any age. The curves close to the fitted line indicate the 95% confidence band for the average acinar volume. As well as this you may well be interested in predicting what the actual acinar volume (as distinct from the average value) would be for a new subject of a specified age. The outer lines (which are symmetrical about the fitted line) indicate the 95% prediction limits and bracket the predicted value in 95 cases out of 100. Note that these are quite wide, a consequence of the considerable biological variability in the data; note also that at age 12 or less the lower prediction limit will be negative, which is clearly impossible. This indicates that a straight line with constant residual variability may not be the most sensible way of fitting these data.

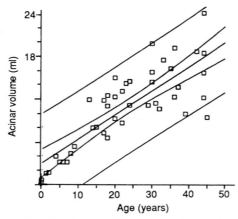

Figure 26 Statgraphics plot of results of linear regression of acinar volume on age. The inner curves indicate the 95% confidence band for the average acinar volume. The outer lines are the 95% prediction limits for actual acinar volume.

Underlying assumptions in regression analysis

In common with other statistical methods, simple linear regression analysis makes several assumptions which should be checked before accepting the results of the analysis. The assumptions are:

(i) the relation is linear;

(ii) the spread of the data about the line is the same at all levels of the explanatory variable;

(iii) the deviations of the data values from the line are normally distributed.

These assumptions can be checked visually with statistical packages by making diagnostic plots of the residuals which are the differences between the observed values of the response variable and the corresponding fitted values. To detect departures from linearity a plot of the residuals against the fitted values is useful. The danger sign is an obvious pattern such as a trend or pronounced curvature.

The same type of plot can be used to detect failure of assumption (ii)—if the points appear to fan out in a wedge then this indicates uneven spread. In either case more advanced techniques of regression analysis may be used to overcome the problem.

A normal plot of the residuals (chapter 2) can be used to check the assumption of normality, although it suffers from the problem that failure of either of the other assumptions can cause the plot to be curved rather than straight. Outliers can also cause problems as they will tend to pull the fitted line towards themselves, particularly if they appear near the extremes of the range of the explanatory variable. Any observation with a particularly large residual should be examined to ensure that it is not erroneous or in some way atypical. Comparing fits with and without suspected outliers will give an indication of their importance in determining the parameters of the line.

In the Minitab package observations which have large residuals or have a large influence on the fitted line are automatically indicated. Statgraphics has similar facilities, including the ability to remove points one at a time and assess the effect of this on the fitted line. If the diagnostic plots indicate that the data do not conform to one or more of the standard assumptions then there are methods for alleviating the problem. If the relation is non-linear then a transformation may provide the remedy. Log transforming either or both the response and explanatory variable(s) may be tried.

The residual plot in fig 27 shows curvature and fanning, indicating that the relation is perhaps curved and that variability

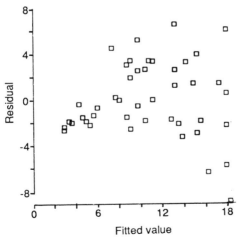

Figure 27   Diagnostic plot of the residuals versus the fitted values for the regression of acinar volume on age. There is a strong pattern (curvature and fanning) which indicates that a linear relation with constant residual variability is not an adequate description of the data.

increases with age. Logarithmic transformation of both variables before fitting a straight line to the log-transformed data is useful here. In this example this leads to the estimated relation:

$$\log(\text{acinar volume}) = 0.356 + 0.49 \times \log(\text{age}),$$

accounting for 86.9% of the variability in the log-transformed volumes. This can then be back-transformed to give the relation:

$$\text{acinar volume} = 2.27 \times \text{age}^{0.49},$$

for which the Statgraphics plot is shown in fig 28. Note that the relation is curved (volume is almost proportional to the square root of age), and that the 95% prediction limits are also curved and diverge with increasing age, which accords more with the pattern of the data.

It must be emphasized that the results of regression analysis can be used validly to predict the size of a response variable for a given value of explanatory variable only within the limits of the range of explanatory variable values used in deriving the regression equation. Any extrapolation is extremely hazardous because it relies on the assumption that the fitted relation holds outside the given range. Acinar volume, for instance, tends to decrease for ages

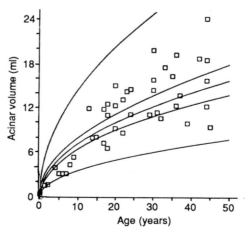

Figure 28   Statgraphics plot of the relation obtained by log-transforming both acinar volume and age before regression analysis. The fitted relation is curved as are the 95% confidence limits (inner curve) and 95% prediction limits (outer curves).

above about 55 years and so neither of the fitted regression equations could be used to predict acinar volumes for ages above 45 years.

The misuse of correlation and regression in method comparison studies

When a new method of measurement is developed it is usual to compare it with the standard method to decide whether it can replace the older method. This is done by making the same measurement by both methods on each of a number of subjects. The important question is whether the measurements agree. Basically the situation is as follows: for each subject there is an unknown true value, so when a measurement is made by a particular method the result will differ from the true value by a measurement error for that particular method. Measurement error varies from one subject to another and is likely to differ between methods. The *precision* of a method is determined by making a number of measurements on the same subject—that is, of the same true value—provided that the true value is stable over the period required to make all the measurements. The standard deviation of the results is a measure of the precision of the method. A method is accurate if the measurements cluster around the true value, and consequently the *accuracy* of a method can only be determined in situations where the true value is known. A series of repeated measurements of the unknown true value for a given subject cannot determine the accuracy of a method.

In comparing two methods of measurement it is important to determine whether they are (a) equally accurate and (b) equally precise. The starting point of the analysis should be a scatter plot of the data as shown in fig 29, which refers to a comparison of measurements of thyroid stimulating hormone concentration (TSH) by radioimmunoassay (RIA) and fluorescence immunoassay (FIA). Note that the "identity line", which has unit slope and zero intercept, is included to provide a guide to interpretation of the plot. Most of the points fall below this line, indicating that the two methods do not agree; note also that there seem to be problems with measurements of low concentrations.

The correlation coefficient is often misused as a way of analysing such data, typically the correlation coefficient will be very high (0·965 in this example) and this is misinterpreted as confirming

65

Figure 29   Scatter plot showing the relation between values obtained by two methods of measurement of thyroid stimulating hormone. Most points fall below the identity line, suggesting a constant proportionate difference between the methods. Some points at low concentrations seem rather erratic.

that the methods agree. This is wrong as the correlation coefficient measures the strength of the relation between the results by the two methods, not whether they tend to agree. A set of measurements which cluster closely around any line, as would occur if one method were to produce results which were on average only 25% of the values given by the other, will result in a high correlation coefficient. As the methods have been developed to measure the same quantity they would be expected to produce measurements which are related.

Closer examination of the problem suggests that methods are likely to disagree in one of two ways: (a) the values will differ on average by a constant amount; (b) the values produced by one method will be on average a fixed percentage of those given by the other—that is, a constant proportionate difference. In case (a) the points will tend to cluster around a line which is parellel to the identity line, whereas in case (b) the points will cluster around a line which has a non-unit slope.

These observations form the basis of a regression method of analysis. If the confidence interval for the slope of the regression line includes the value one then case (b) is eliminated and so the confidence interval for the intercept is examined and if it brackets zero then case (a) is also eliminated and the conclusion is that the methods agree. There is, however, an objection to this method because as both sets of measurements are of unknown true values subject to varying amounts of error there are two regression lines which can be fitted, depending on which method is chosen as the explanatory or x variable. For example, taking RIA as the explanatory variable gives the line;

$$FIA = 0.95 + 0.69 \times RIA$$

with confidence intervals $(0.63, 0.75)$ for the slope and $(-0.01, 1.90)$ for the intercept. Taking FIA as the explanatory variable results in:

$$RIA = -0.47 + 1.36 \times FIA$$

with confidence interval $(1.24, 1.48)$ for slope and $(-1.87, 0.93)$ for intercept. In this case the conclusion is relatively straightforward as neither line is parallel to the identity line, the methods differ by a constant proportionate amount. If one or both methods are imprecise, however, the confidence intervals may be very wide, leading to the possibly erroneous conclusion that the methods agree. In fact, the greater the imprecision the more likely you are to decide that the methods are in agreement using the regression method. With somewhat greater precision the regression method may be equivocal. Take, for example, the case of the hypothetical data illustrated in fig 30. If method A is chosen as the explanatory variable the 95% confidence interval for the slope is $(0.72, 0.95)$, which seems to indicate a constant proportionate difference, but with method B as the explanatory variable the slope confidence interval is $(0.94, 1.24)$ and the intercept interval is $(-30.0, 19.9)$, suggesting that the methods agree.

An extremely simple method of analysis has recently been proposed by Altman and Bland,[15][16] and this is more informative than the regression method. As the differences between corresponding measurements contain the information needed to decide whether the methods agree the most sensible approach is to analyse these differences. To decide between the cases of constant difference and constant proportionate difference, the difference between each pair of measurements is plotted against the average of the pair. If the methods agree then the average of a pair is the best estimate of the corresponding true value and there ought to be no relation between the differences and averages; the scatter plot

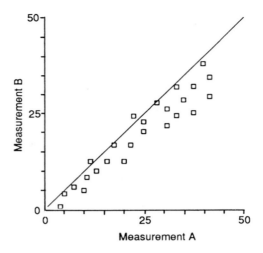

Figure 30   Scatter plot of hypothetical data which produces contradictory results if regression analysis is used in an attempt to assess the degree of agreement between the two methods of measurement.

should show a random cloud of points and the correlation coefficient should not be significant. This will also be true if the methods differ by a constant amount. If the methods differ by a constant proportionate amount, however, then differences between measurements corresponding to large true values will be greater than those corresponding to smaller true values. The plot will then show a significant linear relation with a significant correlation coefficient. This is the case for the TSH comparison (fig 31A).

When methods differ by a constant amount the 95% confidence interval for the mean of the differences indicates the likely size of the difference between the methods. If methods differ by a constant proportionate amount then you should log-transform the raw data and work with the average and difference of the pairs of log-transformed values. When the TSH data are treated in this way most of the points lie in a horizontal band with a few outlying points corresponding to the samples where there were difficulties of measurement at low concentration (fig 31B). The rank correlation, used to attentuate the influence of the outliers, between the differences and averages is 0·17 which is not significant (p > 0·05). The median difference (outliers again) is 0·13 and the distribution free confidence interval (chapter 5) for the median difference

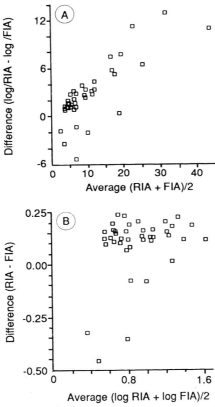

Figure 31 *(A) Differences between individual RIA and FIA values plotted against their averages. There is clearly a linear relation between differences and averages (rank correlation = 0·704, p < 0·01), indicating that there is a constant proportionate difference between the two methods of measurement. (B) Differences between logarithms of individual RIA and FIA values plotted against averages of their logarithms. Most points lie in a horizontal band (rank correlation 0·171, p > 0·1) confirming that there is a constant proportionate difference between the two methods of measurement.*

stretches from 0·10 up to 0·15. Back-transforming this interval we can say that FIA values are likely to be between 71% and 79% of those given by RIA, except at low concentrations where at least one of the methods is very unreliable.

7

Analysis of categorical data

Analysis of counts and proportions

The previous chapters in this book have been concerned with the analysis of data measured on an objective scale ("continuous" data). There are, however, many occasions when some or all of the data are collected as *nominal variables*—that is, something which may fall into one of a set of named categories and is not ordinarily measured—or as *ordinal data*—that is, a feature which can be ranked subjectively by the observer but not measured objectively, as, for example, the severity of an illness. Thus nominal variables arise when each patient may be assigned to one of several mutually exclusive categories distinguished by names—for example, the sex of a patient is either male or female, and there is no meaningful way of ordering such categories. In contrast, an ordinal variable involves a set of mutually exclusive categories which can be sensibly ordered, such as the staging or grading of a neoplasm into categories of increasing extent of disease or greater apparent aggressiveness.

Nominal data may be coded—for example, male = 1, female = 2—but the coding is an arbitrary label because the numerical values chosen as codes have no intrinsic meaning. Ordinal data are commonly coded with the simplest series of ascending integers—for example, none = 0, mild = 1, moderate = 2, severe = 3 —as the integers 0,1,2,3 preserve the relative ordering of the categories, but any other ascending series could be used, as such as none = 0, mild = 6, moderate = 20 and severe = 500. It is essential to remember that the actual increments in the ordinal series (none, mild, moderate, severe) are probably unequal and so when using a coding such as 0,1,2,3 it would be quite improper to assume that "2" was twice as far up the grading scale as "1". It is for this reason that descriptive statistics such as the sample mean and standard deviation should not be used to summarise either nominal or ordinal data (the average sex of a sample of subjects is meaningless).

There are two special situations where data are commonly encountered as counts or proportions. The first concerns measurements using radioactive tracers such as uptake of ^{3}H-TdR as an indicator of DNA synthesis. Here the counts are expressed as counts per minute (cpm) and are often large. The second arises when particular features are counted directly as in enumeration of blood cells or point counting in histometric methods. In both cases relatively large numbers are counted and there will be as many counts or proportions as there are specimens. Consequently, it is often possible to treat the data is if they were true measurements on a continuous scale, but care must be taken to ensure that the data conform to the basic assumptions of the chosen statistical methods of analysis which were devised for measured data.

Estimating a single proportion

It is very unlikely that the sole purpose of an investigation would be the estimation of a single proportion—for example, the proportion of leprosy cases showing the lepromatous form of the disease in a particular country—but it is instructive to look at this example to appreciate some of the limitations of estimation when dealing with proportions. The investigation would proceed by taking a random sample of cases and classifying each one as either lepromatous or not. Thus in 250 cases there might be 175 lepromatous and 75 non-lepromatous so that the estimate (p) of the population proportion would be 175/250 or 0·7. To calculate the 95% confidence interval, as a measure of the precision of this estimate, it is necessary to obtain the standard error of the estimate by substitution of the value of the estimate in the formula:

$$\text{SE of a proportion} = \sqrt{(p(1-p)/n)}$$

and so in this case the standard error is $\sqrt{(0·7 \times 0·3/250)} = 0·029$. The critical value used in calculating the 95% confidence interval is 1·96. By using the formula:

$$\text{estimate} \pm \text{critical value} \times \text{SE of estimate},$$

it is clear that the 95% confidence interval for the proportion of patients with leprosy showing the lepromatous form of the disease stretches from 0·643 up to 0·757, with the usual interpretation that

71

there is a 95% chance that the population percentage could be as low as 64·3% or as high as 75·7%.

This method of calculation of the 95% confidence limits is valid only when the sample size is reasonably large. For very small sample sizes, say 30 or less, the confidence interval can be read directly from a chart given in Neave's tables[12]—for example, if the estimated value of the proportion is 0·7 based on a sample of 10 then Neave's tables give 95% confidence limits stretching from 0·35 up to 0·88. Under these conditions misuse of the formula would give the interval as 0·42 up to 0·98. Notably, the correct interval is not symmetrical about the estimated value of 0·7, but both intervals are so wide as to be virtually useless. This example emphasises how little reliance can be placed on estimates of proportions based on small samples of cases.

One very simple way of assessing the sample size needed to achieve a given precision is to specify the width of confidence interval which is acceptable before the start of the investigation. For example, if the investigator has prior knowledge from reports of similar investigations that the proportion is likely to be around 0·4 and a 95% confidence interval of width 0·1 is required, as the width is twice the critical value multiplied by the standard error of the estimate then:

$$\text{width} = 2 \times 1\cdot96 \times \sqrt{(p(1-p)/n)}.$$

Introducing the prior estimate $p = 0\cdot4$ into this formula results in the equation:

$$0\cdot1 = 3\cdot92 \times \sqrt{(0\cdot24/n)}$$

for which the solution is $n = 369$. This is quite a lot larger than might be anticipated by an inexperienced investigator and shows how much effort is needed to get even moderately precise estimates of proportions.

This calculation requires prior knowledge of the probable size of the proportion which the investigation is supposed to estimate; if it is not possible to make a reasonable guess at this value then $p = 0\cdot5$ should be substituted in the formula relating width to sample size as the standard error takes it maximum value when $p = 0\cdot5$. This gives the simple result:

$$n = (1\cdot96/\text{width})^2$$

for calculating the sample size required for a 95% confidence interval of a given width. This approach will err on the side of caution but will avoid unwarranted optimism in planning investigations.

Comparison of two proportions

It is valid to compare the proportions showing a given character only when the samples have been selected randomly from two populations. In general the sample sizes need not be equal, but it is best if they are not too dissimilar. Bearing in mind the imprecision inherent in estimates of proportions from small samples it would not be sensible to sample 200 subjects from one population and only 20 from the other if a precise estimate of the difference between the proportions was required.

Table 2 gives the results of a comparison of the prevalence of the km1 immunoglobulin allotype in patients with pulmonary tuberculosis and healthy controls in Indonesia. The km1 allotype is present in 32% of the patients and in 57% of the controls. It is more important to determine a confidence interval for the difference between the population proportions than to perform a significance test to determine whether the data provide evidence of a significant difference between the population proportions. The first of these procedures is obviously more informative because it is concerned with practical significance; the second may lead us into the trap of mistakenly emphasising statistical significance.

The χ^2 test is a significance testing procedure which is appropriate in various situations where categorical data must be analysed.[3] In this particular example it provides a test of the hypothesis that the proportion of subjects with the km1 allotype is the same in patients and controls. The test is based on a comparison of what would be expected if this were the case with what is actually

TABLE 2
*Comparison between prevalence of Km1 immunoglobin allotype in
Indonesian patients with pulmonary tuberculosis and healthy controls*

	Km1 positive	Km1 negative	Total
Patients	39	82	121
Controls	72	60	132
Total	111	142	253

observed. As a working hypothesis, suppose that the proportion of subjects with the Km1 allotype is the same in both populations, then the information in the two samples may be combined to give 111/253, or 0·4387 as the best estimate of this proportion. On average, 43·87% of subjects in each sample would be expected to bear the Km1 allotype—that is, 53·08 patients and 57·91 controls—and by similar reasoning 67·92 patients and 74·09 controls would not be expected to carry the Km1 allotype. These are the *expected counts* and they should be interpreted as long run averages; it is clearly impossible to observe fractions of one subject. The overall discrepancy between the observed and expected counts is known as the χ^2 *statistic* and is the sum over the four "cells" of the table of the values of:

$$(\text{observed count} - \text{expected count})^2/\text{expected count}.$$

Regrettably, both Minitab and Statgraphics concentrate on significance testing and ignore estimation. The Minitab output for the χ^2 test is displayed in fig 32. The χ^2 value of 12·765, which has a

```
MTB > NAME C1 'KM1 +'
MTB > NAME C2 'KM1 −'
MTB > CHISQ 'KM1 +' 'KM1 −'

Expected counts are printed below observed counts

            KM1 +   KM1 −    Total
      1       39      82      121
            53·09   67·91

      2       72      60      132
            57·91   74·09

Total        111     142      253

ChiSq =  3·738 + 2·922 +
         3·427 + 2·679 = 12·765
df = 1

MTB > CDF 12·765;
SUBC> CHISQ 1.
   12·7650     0·9996

MTB > NOTE: So the p value is 1 − 0·9996 = 0·0004
```

Figure 32   Minitab output for the χ^2 analysis of incidence of the Km1 immunoglobulin allotype (table 2). CDF command is used to determine the p value of the χ^2 statistic.

p value of 0·0004, indicates that there is extremely strong evidence that the proportion of subjects bearing the Km1 allotype is not the same in the population of patients with pulmonary tuberculosis as it is in the population of healthy controls.

It is a simple matter to produce a table similar to table 2 using Statgraphics. Suppose that the relevant data are stored as two variables, "type" and "Km1", in a file. The "type" variable contains, for each subject, either the value 1 indicating a patient, or the value 2 indicating a control subject. In the same way the "Km1" variable contains, for each subject, either the value 1 indicating a km1 positive test result, or the value 2 indicating a Km1 negative test result. The cross-tabulation option produces a table which shows how many patients and how many controls are Km1 positive and how many are Km1 negative. The input screen setting up the cross-tabulation is shown in fig 33 and this produces the table shown in fig 34. Note that the values below the counts are percentages and not expected counts. A further screen displays the results of the χ^2 test (fig 35). The phrase "with Yates' correction" refers to a particular correction which was originally suggested by the statistician Frank Yates as an attempt to improve the applicability of the χ^2 distribution to the analysis of discrete data. Its use is somewhat controversial as several studies have indicated that it does not always bring about the desired improvement. It is probably best ignored and certainly should not be used as an argument for nudging a marginally significant result in a direction favoured by the investigator.

Statgraphics is less satisfactory than Minitab as it does not give the expected counts. Statgraphics also gives, in the lower half of the display, several statistics which are irrelevant to the problem of

Data vector A:	Km1
Labels A:	2 4 RESHAPE 'Km1 + Km1 − '
Data vector B:	type
Labels B:	2 8 RESHAPE 'patientscontrols'
Percentages:	Rowwise

Figure 33 Input screen to obtain Statgraphics crosstabulation of variables "Km1" and "type". The label fields contain the specification of the labels for individual rows and columns of the table. 2 4 RESHAPE 'Kml1 + Kml −' indicates that the quoted text is to be split into two labels each consisting of four characters. The "rowwise" option has been chosen for percentages, indicating that the values in each row are to be expressed as a percentage of the row total as well as being displayed as row counts.

Cross-tabulation of Km1 by type			
Km1 type	Km1 +	Km1 −	Row Total
patients	39 32·2	82 67·8	121 47·8
controls	72 54·5	60 45·5	132 52·2
Column Total	111 43·9	142 56·1	253 100·0

Figure 34   Cross tabulation of the variables "Km1" and "type" produced by Statgraphics. Note that the lower values in each cell are percentages not expected counts.

Summary Statistics for Contingency Tables			
Chi-Square 12·7651 11·8750	D.F. 1 1	Significance 3·53145E–4 5·68912E–4	with Yates correction
Statistic	Symmetric	With rows dependent	With columns dependent
Lambda	0·14655	0·18182	0·10811
Uncertainty Coeff.	0·03702	0·03684	0·03720
Somer's D	−0·22462	−0·22611	−0·22314
Eta	0·22462	0·22462	0·22462

Figure 35   Statgraphics output for the χ^2 analysis of the Km1 immunoglobulin allotype (table 2). The p value for the test is 0·0004 to four decimal places.

testing whether two population proportions are equal. The various statistics labelled "Lambda", "Uncertainty Coeff", "Somer's D" and "Eta" are all equivalents of the correlation coefficient for counted data and indicate the extent to which the variables used to construct the cross-tabulation are related or associated. This is irrelevant in this particular situation where the question of interest is whether the population proportions differ, and not whether Km1 allotype is related to a subject's status as a patient or a control. To be fair to Statgraphics, the χ^2 test is an "all-purpose test" which can be used to investigate a rather confusing number of different situations, as we shall see, and as the authors of the package can never be sure of the circumstances under which any particular user is applying the test, they have played safe and produced a selection of potentially useful statistics. This illustrates something which the intelligent user of a statistics package should always bear in mind: the fact that certain statistics are automatically produced by the computer does not mean thay are necessarily relevant.

The next and more important step is to calculate a confidence interval so as to interpret the result of the χ^2 test. Unfortunately, neither package does this, but it is quite easy to calculate the 95% confidence interval using the formulae given in the Appendix. The result of the investigation may be summarised as follows: the proportion of patients with pulmonary tuberculosis bearing the km1 allotype is estimated to be 32·3% with a standard error of 4·2%, and for normal controls the proportion is 54·5% with a standard error of 4·3%; this difference is highly significant ($\chi^2 = 12·765$; $p = 0·0004$), and the 95% confidence interval for the difference indicates that the proportion of patients bearing the Km1 allotype is likely to be between 10·4 and 34·2 percentage points lower than the corresponding proportion for healthy controls.

If the sample sizes are very small then a problem may arise. Suppose that we try to analyse the hypothetical data in table 3 which correspond to a drastically scaled down version of the previous investigation. Minitab produces the display shown in fig 36: note the warning message "2 cells with expected counts less than 5·0", which indicates that the sample sizes are too small for the χ^2 test to be reliable. The general rule is that the test is reliable only when all *expected* counts are greater than 5. Note that the rule refers to expected counts, it is quite in order to apply the test when

TABLE 3
Hypothetical results of much smaller investigation of prevalence of Km1 allotype

	Km1 positive	Km1 negative	Total
Patients	2	5	7
Controls	7	6	13
Total	9	11	20

```
MTB > CHISQUARE C1 C2

Expected counts are printed below observed counts
                C1          C2          Total
    1            2           5            7
                3·15        3·85
    2            7           6           13
                5·85        7·15
Total            9          11           20
ChiSq =  0·420 + 0·344 +
         0·226 + 0·185 = 1·174
df = 1
2 cells with expected counts less than 5·0
```

Figure 36   Minitab output for the χ^2 analysis of the data shown in table 3. The warning about expected count less than 5 indicates that the χ^2 test may be misleading.

some observed counts are less than 5, provided that all expected counts exceed 5. There is a test known as *Fisher's exact test* which can be used in this situation and details of which are given in the Appendix. Statgraphics automatically performs the exact test whenever the χ^2 test is likely to be invalid.

The best advice that can be given here is that the investigator should avoid getting into this situation by keeping sample sizes reasonably large. When an investigation aims to compare proportions which are expected to be very small expert advice should be sought as it is likely that extremely large sample sizes will be needed to obtain worthwile data and this may involve multicentre collaboration or data collection over a long period of time. In such circumstances diagnostic criteria, laboratory procedures, and record keeping systems must be carefully standardised, and active quality control of the results, perhaps by means of periodic quality audits will be essential.

Comparison of several proportions

Comparison of several samples from different populations to detect and estimate differences between proportions is dealt with by a straightforward extension of the χ^2 method. The situation is analogous to that in which the analysis of variance is used for measured data, so a single significance test is first applied to all of the data to assess the evidence for any differences beween the samples, and a follow up investigation determines which proportions are different: the problem of multiple comparison analogous to that seen with measured data (chapter 4) arises in the follow up stage.

Table 4 shows the results of Leprosin A skin testing in healthy controls, two groups of patients with leprosy, and two groups of contacts of leprosy victims. The relevant questions here are concerned with whether there are differences between the responsiveness of subjects in the various groups to Leprosin A. The Minitab output is shown in fig 37, with expected counts calculated on the same principle as before; there are a total of 149 positive responses in 253 subjects, so if there were no differences between the rates of positive response in the various subpopulations the best estimate of the common rate of positive responses is 149/253, or 0·589, so 58·9% of each sample might be expected to show a positive skin test and 41·1% to show a negative response. The χ^2 statistic is calculated by summing:

$$(\text{observed count} - \text{expected count})^2 / \text{expected count}$$

for all 10 cells of the table giving the value 16·54, which has a p value of 0·0024. This indicates that the data provide extremely strong evidence of differences between some of the population proportions. To follow up this finding we can calculate a series of multiple confidence intervals for the difference between positive response rates. The details of this procedure are given in the Appendix. Confidence intervals for the differences between positive response rates for each pair of groups are displayed in fig 38, from which it is apparent that the main difference is between hospital contacts of patients with leprosy who have the highest rate of positive response and the group of new patients who have the

TABLE 4
Leprosin A skin tests in various subject groups

| | Test result | | |
	Positive	Negative	Total
Healthy controls (A)	30	20	50
Hospital contacts (B)	18	2	20
Household contacts (C)	45	33	78
Treated patients (D)	35	18	53
New (untreated) patients (E)	21	31	52
Total	149	104	253

```
MTB > NAME C1 'POS.'
MTB > NAME C2 'NEG.'
MTB > CHISQ C1 C2

          Expected counts are printed below observed counts
                    POS.         NEG.         Total
      1              30           20            50
                    29·45        20·55
      2              18            2            20
                    11·78         8·22
      3              45           33            78
                    45·94        32·06
      4              35           18            53
                    31·21        21·79
      5              21           31            52
                    30·62        21·38

   Total            149          104           253

ChiSq = 0·010 + 0·015 +
        3·286 + 4·708 +
        0·019 + 0·027 +
        0·459 + 0·658 +
        3·025 + 4·334 = 16·541
df = 4

MTB > CDF 16·541;
SUBC> CHISQ 4.
   16·5410      0·9976

NOTE: so the p value of the test is 1 − 0·9976 = 0·0024.
```

Figure 37   Minitab output for the χ^2 analysis of the Leprosin A skin test data (table 4). The highly significant χ^2 value indicates that some of the groups differ in responsiveness.

lowest positive response rate. The remaining groups fall in an intermediate position and there are no detectable differences between their response rates.

Multiple category responses

The χ^2 test may also be applied to situations where there are more than two categories of response. Table 5 shows the results of an investigation of the relation between BCG vaccination status and extent of cavitation of the lungs (graded on a four point ordinal scale) in Indonesian patients with pulmonary tuberculosis. The

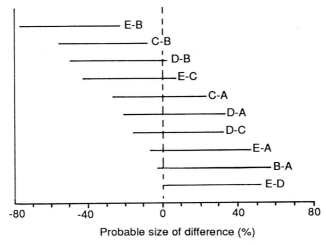

Figure 38 *Multiple comparison confidence intervals for the differences between proportions of positive skin tests for all pairs of groups of subjects. Most of the intervals include zero, indicating that the corresponding pair of groups cannot be regarded as differing in responsiveness. To indicate the groups being compared the lines representing the confidence intervals are labelled with letters assigned to the groups in table 4.*

hypothesis that the underlying distribution of the extent of cavitation does not depend on the vaccination status of the patients is tested by the χ^2 method. A significant result will mean that extent of cavitation does depend on vaccination status. Expected values and the χ^2 statistic are calculated in the same way as in the previous examples and the Minitab output (fig 39A) indicates a problem with small sample sizes as one expected count is considerably less than 5. This may be dealt with by combining the first two

TABLE 5
Relation between BCG vaccination status and cavitation of lung in Indonesian patients with pulmonary tuberculosis

Extent of cavitation	Vaccinated	Not vaccinated	Total
0	4	31	35
1	4	9	13
2	13	18	31
3	3	27	30
Total	24	85	109

```
MTB > CHISQ C1 C2
              Expected counts are printed below observed counts
                         C1          C2         Total
        1                 4          31           35
                        7·71       27·29

        2                 4           9           13
                        2·86       10·14

        3                13          18           31
                        6·83       24·17

        4                 3          27           30
                        6·61       23·39

    Total                24          85          109

ChiSq = 1·783 + 0·503 +
        0·452 + 0·128 +
        5·585 + 1·577 +
        1·968 + 0·556 = 12·551
df = 3
1 cells with expected counts less than 5·0
```

```
MTB > CHISQ C1 C2

              Expected counts are printed below observed counts
                         C1          C2         Total
        1                 8          40           48
                       10·57       37·43

        2                13          18           31
                        6·83       24·17

        3                 3          27           30
                        6·61       23·39

    Total                24          85          109

ChiSq = 0·624 + 0·176 +
        5·585 + 1·577 +
        1·968 + 0·556 = 10·486
df = 2
MTB > CDF 10·486;
SUBC> CHISQ 2.
    10·4860      0·9947

NOTE: So the p value of the test is 1 − 0·9947 = 0·0053.
```

Figure 39 *(A) Minitab output for the data relating extent of lung cavitation to BCG vaccination status (table 5). One of the expected counts is less than 5, so the χ^2 test could be misleading. (B) By combining results for adjacent cavitation grades (0,1) the expected counts are raised to permit valid use of the χ^2 test.*

cavitation categories (cavitation index none or one) to obtain higher expected counts. This leads to the analysis shown in fig 39B, from which we conclude that extent of cavitation is not independent of BCG vaccination status. The main difference between the distributions of extent of cavitation seems to be a relative excess of cavitation grade 3 (cavities in two lung zones) among the BCG vaccinated patients. Interpretation of this type of investigation is necessarily more complex as you are looking for differences in the overall pattern of the multiple category grading variable and such differences cannot be summarised in terms of one or two simply interpretable numbers.

Point or structure counts, radioactive counts

Where an investigation entails direct counts of structures in tissue sections or estimation of proportionate areas or volumes occupied by various features then although the end result will be expressed as a proportion, the method of analysis to be used is quite different from that described in the earlier sections of this chapter. The same will be true of investigations which use radioactive cpm as an indirect method of measuring some aspect of cellular activity, such as DNA synthesis. The essential difference is that each case will result in a separate proportion or count rather than contributing a small amount. In this case proportions and cpm can be treated as if they were measurements and all of the methods appropriate to measured data may be used after suitable transformation of the data.

Proportions and cpm, however, are not true measurements and they do not conform to all the assumptions that the standard methods devised for continuous data require for their validity. In particular, the assumption of constant residual variability is not met. The variability in a set of proportions is related to the size of the proportions, thus small and large proportions have less scope for being variable because they cannot extend beyond zero or unity, whereas the intermediate proportions have more room for variability. To nullify this effect proportions should, in this situation, always be transformed by means of the angular transformation[3] (also known as the arc-sine transformation) before methods such as analysis of variance or regression analysis are applied.

From the theory of radiation physics it can be shown that

radioactive counts conform to the Poisson distribution, not the normal distribution. One of the important consequences of this is that the variability of radioactive cpm will be directly proportional to their average. In this situation the raw data must be transformed by taking square roots of counts before applying analysis of variance or regression methods.

Appendix

Expected counts and degrees of freedom

There is a simple rule for calculating the expected counts for each cell of the table:

$$\text{expected count} = \text{row total} \times \text{column total}/\text{grand total}.$$

The degrees of freedom associated with the χ^2 statistic are equal to one less than the number of rows in the table multiplied by one less than the number of columns.

Confidence intervals

The standard error of the estimate (p) of a proportion is $\sqrt{(p(1-p)/n)}$ and the confidence interval is:

$$\text{estimate} \pm \text{critical value} \times \text{SE of estimate}$$

The critical value is 1·96 for a 95% interval, 2·58 for a 99% interval, and 2·81 for a 99·5% interval. These critical values are the upper 2·5%, 0·5%, and 0·25% points of the normal distribution.

If the estimates of two proportions are p_1 and p_2 based on samples of sizes n_1 and n_2 then the standard error of their difference is:

$$\sqrt{(p_1(1-p_1)/n_1 + p_2(1-p_2)/n_2)}$$

and a confidence interval for the difference between the proportions is:

$$(p_1 - p_2) \pm \text{critical value} \times \text{SE of difference},$$

the same critical values being used.

Multiple comparison of a set of proportions

The confidence intervals shown in fig 38 were calculated by applying the formula for the confidence interval for the difference between two proportions to all possible pairs of proportions. To maintain an overall error rate of 5% in the complete set of comparisons the confidence coefficient of each interval must be 100%–5%/(number of comparisons). In the example there are 10 comparisons so the confidence coefficient must be 99·5% and each interval will be of the form:

$$\text{difference} \pm 2{\cdot}81 \times \text{SE of difference.}$$

For example, the proportion of positive skin tests among the hospital controls is 0·9 and among the healthy controls it is 0·6. The difference is 0·3 with a standard error equal to $\sqrt{(0{\cdot}6 \times 0{\cdot}4/50) + (0{\cdot}9 \times 0{\cdot}1/20))}$, or 0·096 so the confidence interval is 0·3 ± 2·81 × 0·096 or 0·3 ± 0·27, (30% ± 27%). Note that a separate calculation of the standard error is needed for each pair of groups being compared.

Fisher's exact text

The exact test calculates the p value associated with the observed table on the hypothesis that there is no difference between the corresponding population proportions. This is done by summing the probability of occurrence of the observed table and all tables which have the same marginal totals but are more extreme than it is. In the example these are the tables shown in fig 40, which are obtained by putting 0,1 and 2 in the upper top left corner. This then determines the remaining three entries because the row and column totals are fixed.

If O_1, O_2, O_3, and O_4 denote the values in the body of the table, R_1, R_2, C_1, C_2, and N the row totals, column totals, and grand total, respectively, then the probability associated with this particular table is:

$$\frac{R_1! \times R_2! \times C_1! \times C_2!}{N! \times O_1! \times O_2 \times O_3! \times O_4!}$$

where, for example R_1 ! (read as "R_1 factorial") is the product of the integers from 1 up to R_1, (in this example $R_1 = 7$ and

0	7	7		1	6	7		2	5	7
9	4	13		8	5	13		7	6	13
9	11	20		9	11	20		9	11	20

Figure 40   The p value of Fisher's exact test is calculated by summing the probabilities of occurrence associated with these three tables (derived from table 3).

$7! = 7 \times 6 \times 5 \times 4 \times 3 \times 2 \times 1$ or 5040). Note also that the numerical value of 0! (zero factorial) is 1.

The probabilities associated with the three tables in fig 40 are

$(7! \times 13! \times 9! \times 11!)/(20! \times 7! \times 9! \times 4!)$,
$(7! \times 13! \times 9! \times 11!)/(20! \times 1! \times 6! \times 8! \times 5!)$ and
$(7! \times 13! \times 9! \times 11!)/(20! \times 2! \times 5! \times 7! \times 6!)$ or 0·004, 0·053, and 0·215, so the p value of the observed table is 0·272, leading to the conclusion that observed results provide no evidence of a difference between the proportions.

8

Statistical methods for diagnostic tests

Reference ranges

Most tests used in clinical medicine give a numerical result on a continuous measurement scale. The pathologists or clinicians attempt to interpret the result by comparing it with a "reference range" previously calculated from a study of people who do not have the disease in question. By current convention, the reference range includes all but the top and bottom 2·5% of the results expected from a population of healthy people, so that 5% of the "normal" healthy population will have test values falling outside the reference range. Consequently, the fact that the test result for an individual subject is outside the reference range does not necessarily imply that the individual is abnormal—this is one reason why the older term "normal range" is becoming obsolete.

A reference range may be determined from test values obtained from a sample of healthy subjects, provided (i) the subjects constitute a random sample from the healthy portion of the population and (ii) the sample size is sufficiently large for it to be representative of the population and for the sample mean and standard deviation to be precise estimates of the population mean and standard deviation.

If the population distribution of the test results is normal, then 95% of all values will lie within the range:

population mean ± 1·96 (population standard deviation)

(chapter 2). The sample mean and standard deviation are estimates of the unknown population mean and standard deviation and by convention the *reference range* is taken to be:

sample mean ± 1·96 (sample standard deviation)

The sample mean and standard deviation are, however, subject to sampling variation—that is, each random sample gives rise to different sample statistics—and so the limits of the reference range will be imprecise. Confidence intervals can be calculated for the upper and lower reference limits to indicate the imprecision of the reference range. If the sample size is large a 95% confidence interval for each end of the reference range is:

$$\text{reference limit} \pm 1\cdot96\sqrt{3} \ (\text{SE mean}).$$

The method for calculation can be illustrated by data obtained in a study of the prevalence and titre of IgE antibodies to *Mycobacterium tuberculosis* in healthy Indonesian factory workers (group A, fig 41). The distribution of the counts in the radioallergosorbent test (RAST) is not symmetrical but it becomes so after logarithmic transformation. These log-transformed results have a reference range of 1·42 to 3·20; the 95% confidence interval calculation indicates that the upper limit for the upper end of the range is 3·28 and the lower limit for the lower end point is 1·34. If these limits are back-transformed (using antilogs) this results in a reference range of 22 to 1905 cpm.

The concept of a reference range is not restricted to medical diagnosis but appears in the guise of a "tolerance interval" in industrial quality control. Comprehensive information on the internationally accepted definition of a statistical tolerance interval is contained in ISO Standard 3207.[17] The validity of the calculations of the reference range and the confidence intervals for the reference limits depends very critically on the assumption that the test values are normally distributed so the sample must be assessed for normality and possible outliers using methods described in chapter 2 before starting the reference range calculation. If the data are not normally distributed or contain inexplicable outliers the sample mean and standard deviation method cannot be used to determine the reference range. If the data are skewed to the right, a square root or a logarithmic transformation (as used with the data of fig 41) may bring about symmetry and perhaps normality, thus allowing calculation by the above method.

Usually it will be safer to determine reference limits by a method which does not require normality of the raw test results. A universally applicable method is based on the percentiles of the observed distribution of the sample values. Any given percentile is that value below which a specified percentage of the distribution lies; so 2·5% of the sample values do not exceed the 2·5 percentile

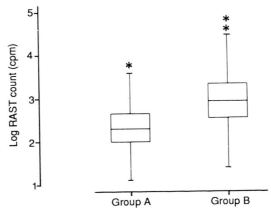

Figure 41   Box and whisker plots comparing titre of IgE antibodies to Mycobacterium tuberculosis using the radioallergosorbent test (RAST) in 350 healthy Indonesian factory workers (group A) and 350 Indonesian tuberculosis patients (group B). Both distributions are symmetrical on a logarithmic scale. Group A: mean of log counts = 2·31, SD of log counts = 0·45. Group B: mean of log counts = 2·96, SD of log counts = 0·58.

and 97·5% of sample values do not exceed the 97·5 percentile (this is analogous to the quartiles introduced in chapter 2). On condition that the sample size is sufficiently large, this provides a very simple method of determining reference limits. Statgraphics will automatically calculate any specified percentiles of a set of results and for the test results of the healthy workers shown in fig 41 the 2·5 and 97·5 percentiles of the untransformed RAST counts are 26 and 1518. This technique will only produce reliable results if the sample size is sufficiently large for the sample to be representative of the variability in the population (greater than 100 to be safe). For small samples the sample percentiles will be very imprecise estimates of the corresponding population values. A 95% confidence interval for the 2·5 percentile may be found as follows: first calculate,

$$0.025 \text{ (sample size)} \pm 1.96\sqrt{(0.025 \times 0.975 \times \text{sample size})}$$

This will give two values which will not usually be integers: then round the values up to the next integer.[18] For example, if the sample size is 350 then the above calculation gives the values 3·48 and 14·02 which are rounded up to 4 and 15. This means that the 95% confidence interval for the 2·5 percentile stretches from the

89

4th smallest up to the 15th smallest test value (17 to 32). The corresponding interval for the 97·5 percentile is determined by counting down the same number of values from the largest test value (giving 1180 to 1995). Thus the reference range based on percentiles, and allowing for uncertainty in the percentiles, is 17 to 1995, which is not very different from that found by using the previous method based on the assumption of normality of log RAST count.

There are several sources of variation which are likely to affect the test value produced by any well monitored and accurately calibrated analytical technique for a given subject. For example (a) inherent random error in the analysis of the sample, usually monitored by quality control methods, (b) time-related variation, (c) variation associated with physiological changes, (d) variation associated with external factors such as diet, tobacco, or alcohol consumption, exercise, posture, and so on, before taking the test specimen. Such factors will tend to increase the variability of results and, in the absence of information about the magnitude of their effects on variability it may be difficult to interpret a result which lies "just outside" the reference range. Thus a healthy subject who has a "true" value close to the upper reference limit may give a test result above the limit. Similarly, a diseased subject who has a "true" value above the upper reference limit could be within the reference range when tested.

Assessment of diagnostic tests

In view of the uncertainties inherent in comparing a test result with a reference range it is worth while examining the criteria that should be used in assessing and choosing diagnostic tests.[19] [20] To assess a particular diagnostic method results must first be obtained from a group of subjects who have the fully developed disease and a group in which the disease is absent. In practice, diagnostic tests are often used to assess patients who are in the early stages of disease; this raises the issue of whether comparison of the above groups addresses the correct question. The criteria for determining the presence and absence of the disease in these two groups must be carefully stated and should agree with standard well understood and accepted methodology (a "gold" standard). The criteria for what constitutes a positive test result must be carefully and unambiguously stated. For example, if the test result is determined by comparison of peaks on a chart then the precise way in which the peaks are located and exactly how they are compared should be explained unambiguously.

If the initial studies on a proposed new diagnostic method were based on 350 healthy subjects and 350 patients with pulmonary tuberculosis patients who have been diagnosed as having the disease on the basis of some independent, well defined, and accepted criterion (in this case chest x ray pictures), the test results might be as shown in fig 41. The investigator might perform a Mann-Whitney test (chapter 5), as the test results are not normally distributed, the resulting p value being less than 0·0001.

The investigator would be wrong to conclude from this that the assay has high diagnostic value because the Mann-Whitney test is designed to answer the question, "do the data provide evidence of a difference in the medians of the population distributions for healthy and diseased persons?" This is largely irrelevant for judging the clinical value of a diagnostic test, where the critical decision *must* involve a notion of a cut off point to assist in decision taking. In practice, values above a certain critical limit will be regarded as indicating that the patient has the disease and lower values that it is unlikely that the patient has the disease. The pertinent question must concern not merely the separation between the medians (or means) of the corresponding population distributions for the healthy and diseased groups but separation of the distributions *as a whole*. It is relatively common for the distributions to overlap (fig 8), and this raises the possibility that a healthy subject will be classified as diseased or that a diseased subject may be classified as healthy. Assessment of a diagnostic test must concentrate on such issues and look at the risks of misclassification.

As the initial assessment of the value of the proposed new test depends on its application to a group of patients with clearly established disease and to people who are undoubtedly healthy the results for any selected cut off point can be summarised in a 2×2 table as shown in fig 42. The *sensitivity* of a test is defined as the proportion of the patients who have the disease in whom the test result is positive $(a/(a+c))$, and this is a measure of the probability that a person who has the disease will give a positive test result. The *specificity* of a test is defined as the proportion of healthy subjects in whom the test result is negative, $(d/(b+d))$, and this measures the probability that a healthy person will give a negative

		disease present	absent	Total
Test	positive	a	b	a+b
Result	negative	c	d	c+d
	Total	a+c	b+d	a+b+c+d

Figure 42   For any specified cut off point the results of a single test on a group of patients with the disease and a group of controls without the disease may be classified into a 2 × 2 table.

test result. The *false positive rate* is the proportion of healthy subjects who give a positive test result $(b/(b+d))$, and the *false negative rate* is the proportion of subjects who have the disease but give a negative result $(c/(a+c))$. Thus in this example with the cut off point set at an RAST count of 320 the test correctly identified 71·4% of those with the disease, but failed to detect the disease in 28·6% of cases. It also correctly identified 72·6% of those who were disease free but was positive in 27·4% of cases where the disease was absent (fig 43).

Very few diagnostic tests have 100% sensitivity and 100% specificity and consequently it should be realised that although knowledge of these operating characteristics of a test are very important, this is not in itself sufficient to determine the probability that the disease is present when the test result is positive, or of absence when the test proves negative.

When selecting a test it is necessary to compare the sensitivity and specificity of the available tests. As a general rule, the test with the highest sensitivity should be selected for clinical diagnosis unless its specificity is unacceptably low. When a test is to be

		disease present	absent	Total
Test	positive	250	96	346
Result	negative	100	254	354
	Total	350	350	700

Figure 43   The observed incidence of positive and negative test results based on the data of figure 41 when a positive result is defined as a RAST count exceeding 320 cpm.

applied for screening purposes it can be argued that it is important that as large a proportion as possible of thòse who give a positive test result do, in fact, have the disease the screening program is meant to detect, and so the sensitivity should be high. A test used to confirm a diagnosis should have a high specificity—that is, it should produce a negative result in a high proportion of those who do not have the disease.

The sensitivity and specificity of a test can be changed by altering the criterion for positivity. When the test gives numerical values on a continuous scale a cut off point is used to define the boundary between positive and negative results—for example, in fig 41 a cut off point at 500 (log 500 = 2·699) results in a sensitivity of 66% and a specificity of 77%. By moving the cut off point down the scale a greater proportion of diseased subjects will give a positive test result so the sensitivity increases, but this occurs at the cost of fewer subjects without the disease giving a negative result—that is, decreasing specificity. The *receiver-operator characteristic (ROC) curve* of a test is a graph which is constructed by plotting, for a series of cut off points, the sensitivity (true positive rate) against the false positive rate (100-specificity). This curve is shown in fig 44 for the data displayed in fig 41, and it is apparent that the test cannot provide a very high true positive rate coupled with a low false positive rate. The ROC may be used to determine the

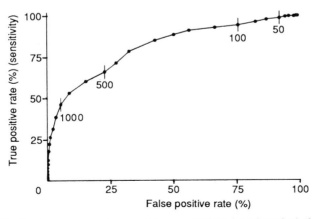

Figure 44   Receiver-operator characteristic curve (ROC) for a hypothetical diagnostic test based on the RAST counts of figure 41. Selected cut off points are marked.

optimal cut off point for the test according to the costs and benefits (in the widest sense) resulting from correct and incorrect diagnoses. Competing tests may be assessed by comparing their ROC curves.

The probability that a patient with a positive test result has the disease depends not only on the sensitivity and specificity of the test but also on the pre-test or prior estimate of the probability that a patient presenting with a particular combination of signs and symptoms has the disease. Note that an investigation designed to assess a test and determine its ROC curve does not provide this information because the assessment will be based on approximately equal numbers of healthy and diseased subjects. The prior estimate of disease probability must be based on past experience of the prevalence of the disease among patients with the specified signs and symptoms.

If the prior estimate was—for example, 50%—that is, in 2000 patients presenting 1000 would be expected to have the disease—then the data from the test evaluation may be combined with this information to give the results shown in fig 45. Of the 1000 patients with the disease, 714 will give a positive test result and 274 of the 1000 patients who do not have the disease will also be positive. Consequently, 988 positive test results would be expected, and the proportion of diseased patients among these is 714 out of 988 or 72·3%. Thus a positive test result converts a 50% chance that the patient has the disease into a 72% chance. The *positive predictive value* (PPV) of a positive test result is the probability that a patient who gives a positive test has the disease and the *predictive value of a negative result* (PVN) is the corresponding probability that a patient with a negative result does not have the disease. Table 6 shows the positive and negative predictive value for prior estimates

| | | disease | | Total |
		present	absent	
Test	positive	714	274	988
Result	negative	286	726	1022
Total		1000	1000	2000

Figure 45 Expected numbers of subjects in the four categories in a group of 2000 subjects if a positive test result is defined as a RAST count exceeding 320 cpm, when the prior estimate of the disease probability is 0·5.

TABLE 6

Prior estimate of disease probability	Positive predictive value	Predictive value of a negative result
0·1	0·225	0·958
0·3	0·528	0·856
0·5	0·723	0·717
0·7	0·859	0·521
0·9	0·959	0·220

ranging from 10% to 90% when the sensitivity and specificity of the test are 71·4% and 72·6%. In this case the results are not particularly impressive, which is a reflection of the fact that the RAST count is not a good diagnostic indicator in this particular situation.

It must be borne in mind that the results of an assessment of a diagnostic test, which compares those without the disease and those with fully developed disease, are likely to overstate the predictive value of a positive or a negative result when the test is applied to patients who do not have the fully developed disease because the distribution of test results in such patients is likely to be closer to that of the disease free group than the distribution of test results from patients with fully developed disease.

Discriminant analysis

There are many clinical situations in which a single diagnostic test may not be sufficiently specific or sensitive to diagnose a disease and it is usual to perform two or more different tests and base the diagnosis on the combined results. The assessment of such situations leads naturally to investigation of the sensitivity and specificity of the combination of two or more tests. *Discriminant analysis* is the method generally chosen for determining objectively the cut off region between controls and patients. For example, assays for serum factor VIII based on radioimmunoassay and bioassay were compared for their diagnostic value in detecting women who were carriers of haemophilia.[21] The results for each test taken separately showed substantial overlap between women who were carriers and controls. When, however, the results were displayed in a scatterplot, it was clear that the two groups could be separated almost completely by an imaginary diagonal line (fig 46). On this basis it

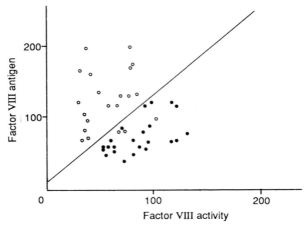

Figure 46   *Scatterplot of the results of radioimmunoassay (antigen) and bioassay (activity) of serum factor VIII in 21 definite female carriers of haemophilia (○) and 23 normal women (●). The straight line indicates the linear discriminant function.*

would be possible to set out the rule, "classify the subject as a carrier if the results of the pair of tests lie above the line." For this cut off line the sensitivity is 86% and the specificity is 100%, so the combination of the two tests is an immense improvement over the use of either test alone.

Discriminant analysis[22][23] is the name given to the statistical technique for determining objectively the position of the line which best discriminates between the two groups, in the sense of producing as few misclassifications as possible in the data from the original investigation. The line separating the two groups defines the *linear discriminant function* which is merely a formula for combining both test results into a single *discriminant score* which may then be used to assess sensitivity and specificity in the usual way. The Statgraphics output for the data of fig 46 is shown in fig 47, the "unstandardised discriminant function coefficients" are interpreted in the following way: for each of the 44 women calculate:

$$0{\cdot}0347(\text{factor VIII antigen}) - 0{\cdot}0272(\text{factor VIII activity}) + 0{\cdot}2853,$$

this is the discriminant score for each woman. Whether a person is classified by *the data alone* as a carrier or as normal depends on

Discriminant analysis for factor VIII
Unstandardised Discriminant Function Coefficients

	1
activity	0·0347
antigen	− 0·0272
CONSTANT	0·2853

Figure 47 Statgraphics output for linear discriminant analysis of the data of figure 46.

whether her score is positive or negative; negative scores are indicative of carrier status. Obviously, anyone with a zero score cannot be classified and this fact allows the discriminating line to be drawn. We may rewrite this condition as discriminant score = 0 or as:

$$0·0272(\text{factor VIII activity}) = 0·0347(\text{factor VIII antigen}) + 0·2853,$$

On dividing throughout by 0·0272 this becomes:

$$\text{factor VIII activity} = 1·28(\text{factor VIII antigen}) + 10·50,$$

which is the equation of the straight line drawn in fig 46. The discriminant score for any subject is related to the perpendicular distance from this line to the point corresponding to her activity and antigen results.

The discrimination is not perfect; three of the known carriers are misclassified as normal. The overall misclassification rate of 3 out of 21 carriers and 0 out of 23 normal controls is bound to be somewhat overoptimistic as an estimate of what is likely to happen if the rule is used in future, because the discriminant function is designed to minimise the total proportion of those who are misclassified for the available data. The discriminant scores for both groups are plotted in fig 48 and show almost complete separation of the groups.

The sensitivity and specificity of the pair of tests may be examined by calculating the misclassification rates for other cut off points than that resulting from the discriminant analysis. This is done by replacing the constant in the discriminant score (0·2853) by a range of alternatives. The data manipulation facilities of Statgraphics can be used to calculate the discriminant score 0·0347(factor VIII antigen) − 0·0272(factor VII activity) for each

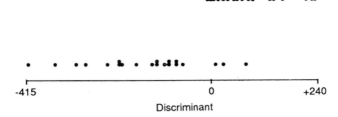

-415   0   +240

Discriminant

Figure 48   Plot of the discrimination scores for the data of figure 46.

person in both the control and the carrier group and the tabulation facilities can be used to calculate how many subjects of either group have a discriminant score less than each alternative cut off value, and from this the sensitivity and specificity at each alternative value can be determined which enables the ROC curve to be plotted.

Discriminant analysis is not limited to pairs of measurements, it may be applied to situations where several different measurements have been made on each of several subjects in different groups with the intention of finding linear discriminant functions which allow newly observed subjects to be allocated to one of the groups. It should be noted, however, that the method will be reliable only if the subjects used in the original investigation were allocated to the groups by some well understood and reliable method.

The method of discriminant analysis used by Statgraphics and similar packages cannot cope successfully with data which consist of a mixture of measurements (continuous variables) and categorical or ordinal data. Advice from your local statistical guru should be sought if your data include both types of variables.

Reprise

This book has presented several standard techniques of statistical analysis and has sought to emphasise the importance of using statistical analysis to answer the *right* questions. It will be apparent from the discussion of the misuse of correlation and regression in comparison of laboratory methods and in the discussion on the evaluation of diagnostic tests in this chapter that it is sometimes easy to lose sight of the questions central to the scientist's investigations in the search for a convenient statistical technique. The investigator should always remember that it is stupid to use the wrong technique to answer an irrelevant question. This situation can be avoided by asking several questions at the beginning of the investigation:

(a) What is the precise aim of the investigation?

(b) If a very large amount of a particular type of data were available, would they provide the answer to the questions being asked?

(c) Is the investigation concerned with differences or similarities between groups?

(d) Is the investigation large enough to detect clinically important differences?

Finally, you should attempt to clear your mind of the idea that all that is important is the calculation of some result (any result) which has a p value small enough to allow the result to be declared "significant". Many statistical text books with a heavy emphasis on statistical significance testing do not help in this respect. At the risk of boring the reader we will reiterate our view that statistical significance should always be related to clinical or biological importance, and a full measure of common sense (with clinical or scientific insight) should be exercised in planning an investigation and interpreting its results.

Acknowledgements

We are grateful to the former editor of the *Journal of Clinical Pathology*, Professor G Slavin, for commissioning these articles, to Ms Caroline White for helpful editorial advice, to Mr R S Fawkes and Dr J H Gibbs for assistance in the preparation of the figures, to Miss M C K Browning of the Department of Biochemical Medicine, Ninewells Hospital and Medical School, for allowing us to use the data on TSH assays in chapter 6, and to Professor C D Forbes of the Department of Medicine, University of Dundee, for giving us access to the data used in chapter 8 on factor VIII concentrations in women who may be carriers of haemophilia.

References

1 Pocock SJ. *Clinical trials: a practical approach.* New York: John Wiley and Sons, 1983.
2 Gore S, Altman DG. *Statistics in practice.* London: British Medical Association, 1982.
3 Armitage P. *Statistical methods in medical research.* Oxford: Blackwell Scientific Publications, 1971.
4 Bailey NTJ. *Statistical methods in biology.* London: Hodder and Stoughton, 1981.
5 Ingelfinger JA, Mosteller F, Thibodeau LA, Ware JH. *Biostatistics in clinical medicine.* 2nd ed. New York: Macmillan, 1987.
6 Diem K, Lentner C, eds. *Documenta Geigy, Scientific tables.* Basle: Geigy, 1970.
7 Gardner MJ, Altman DG. Confidence intervals rather than p values: estimation rather than hypothesis testing. *Br Med J* 1986;**292**:746–50.
8 Rothman K. A show of confidence. *N Engl J Med* 1978;**299**:1362–3.
9 Miller RG. *Simultaneous statistical inference* New York: Springer-Verlag, 1981.
10 Conover WJ. *Practical non-parametric statistics.* New York: John Wiley and Sons, 1980.
11 Sprent P. *Quick statistics.* London: Penguin, 1981.
12 Neave HR. *Elementary statistics tables.* London: Allen and Unwin, 1981.
13 Kowalski CJ. On the effects of non-normality on the distribution of the sample product moment correlation coefficient. *Applied Statistics* 1972;**21**:1–12.
14 Gayen AK. The frequency distribution of the product moment correlation coefficient in samples of any size drawn from non-normal universes. *Biometrika* 1951;**38**:219–47.
15 Altman DG, Bland JM. Measurement in medicine: the analysis of method comparison studies. *Statistician* 1983;**32**:307–17.
16 Bland JM, Altman DG. Statistical methods for assessing agreement between two methods of clinical measurement. *Lancet* 1986;i:307–10.
17 International Standards Organisation. *Statistical tolerance intervals, ISO standards 3207.* Geneva:ISO, 1980.
18 Conover WJ. *Practical nonparametric statistics.* New York: John Wiley and Sons, 1980:111–6.
19 Griner PF, Mayewski RJ, Mushlin AI, Greenland P. Selection and interpretation of diagnostic tests and procedures: principles and applications. *Ann Intern Med* 1981;**94**:553–600.
20 Anonymous. When is a test diagnostic? [Editorial.] *Hum Pathol* 1985;**16**:325.
21 Prentice CRM, Forbes CD, Morrice S, McLaren AD. Calculation of predictive odds for possible carriers of haemophilia. *Thromb Diath Haem* 1975;**34**:740–7.
22 Fisher RA. The use of multiple measurements in taxonomic problems. *Ann Eugenics* 1936;**7**:179–88.
23 Morrison DF. *Multivariate statistical methods.* Tokyo: Kogakusha/McGraw-Hill:1976:230–45.

Index

Accuracy   4, 65
Altman and Bland method   67
Analysis of variance   35
  basic principle   36
  distribution free   48–49
  follow up analysis   37–39
  replicas and repeated measures
    41–42
  residuals   39–40
Angular transformation (arc-sine)
  83

BASIC program   50
Box and whisker plot   13–15, 32,
  34, 45

Categorical data   70–84
  multiple responses   80–83
Chi-squared test   73
  interpretation of results   77–78
  statistic   74
  "with Yates' correction"   75
Command lines   10
Comparative investigations
  paired comparison   29, 47
  several groups   34–42
  two sample   26–29, 44
Confidence intervals   24–25,
  27–29
  compared with significance
    tests   29–33
Correlation coefficient   52–55
  misuse   65
  rank   56
Counts   70–71
  expected   74

radioactive   83–84
  structure   83

Data
  continuous   9
  entering   1–3, 7
  nominal   9, 70
  ordinal   9, 70
  transformation   14, 43, 44
Database management systems   3
Diagnostic plots   39–40, 62–64
Diagnostic tests
  assessment   90–95
  discriminant analysis   95–98
  false negative rate   92
  false positive rate   92
  positive predictive value   94
  receiver-operator curve   93–94
  reference ranges   87–90
  sensitivity and specificity   91
Discriminant analysis   95–98
Displays   11
  to avoid   14–16
Distribution
  normal   17
  poisson   84
  symmetrical   17
  unimodal   17
Distribution free methods   43
  analysis of variance   48–49
  assumptions   44, 48
  t test equivalent   44–48
Dot plot   11–12, 32

Error rate   35
Experimental investigations   5–6

False negative rate   92
False positive rate   92
Fisher's exact test   77–78, 85
Follow up analysis   37–39

Graphical displays   11

Histogram   12
Human variation   4–5

Importing   10
Interquartile range   13
Investigations
  comparative   26–29
  experimental   5–6
  observational   6
ISO Standard 3207   88

Kruskal-Wallis test   48–49

Linear regression analysis   57–61
  assumptions   62–65
  discriminant function   96
  method comparison   67
  model   58
Lotus 123 (Spreadsheet)   2

Mann-Whitney
  procedure   44–47, 91
Mean and error bar plot   14–15
Measurement
  comparison of methods   65–69
  error   65
Menu system   8
Methods of measurement
  comparison   65–69
  correlation   65–66
  regression analysis   66
  source of variability   4
Minitab   7, 10, 25, 45, 47, 54, 57,
  63, 79
  analysis of variance   38
  chi-squared test   74, 77
Missing values   9–10
Monotonic curve   56
Multiple comparisons procedure
  39
Multivariate analysis   42

Neave's tables   72
Nominal data   9, 70
Normal distribution   16–19
Normal plotting   18

Observational studies   6
Ordinal data   9, 70
Outliers   16, 63

Point counts   83
Population
  defining   20–21
  mean   17, 21, 24–25, 27
  standard deviation   22–24
Predictive values   94
Precision   4, 65
Probability level   25, 32
Product-moment correlation
  coefficient   52
Proportions
  several compared   78–80
  single   71–73
  two-compared   73–78

Radioactive counts   82–83
Randomisation   5
Rank correlation   56
Receiver-operator characteristic
  curve   93–94
Reference ranges   87–90
  limits   88–89
  sources of variation   90
Repeated measures   42
Replicates   41
Residuals   39–40, 62–64

Sample
  mean   24
  standard deviation   24
Sampling   4
  distribution of the mean   24
Scatter plots   52–53, 66–68
Significance tests   29, 37
  basis   30
  chi-squared test   73
  shortcomings   30–31
  spurious significance   40, 57
  with confidence intervals   32
Spreadsheet programs   1

repetitive values   2–3
  using   2
Standard deviations   13
  population   22, 23
  sample   24
Standard error of mean   16,
  24–25
Statgraphics   3, 7, 10, 12, 18, 32,
  39, 47, 53, 57
  analysis of variance   37
  chi-squared test   75–77
  linear regression analysis   59,
  61, 64
  main menu   8
Statistical packages   6–8
  data entry facilities   3
Structure counts   83
Summary statistics
  magnitude   12–13
  spread   13
  symmetry   14

t tests   30
Tolerance interval   88

Transformation of data   14,
  43–44, 64, 68

Variability
  replicates   41
  sources   4–5
Variables
  correlation   52–57, 65
  explanatory   57
  linear regression
  analysis   57–65
  misuse of correlation and
  regression   65
  nominal   70
  ordinal   70
  response   57
Variance *See* Analysis of variance

Wilcoxon technique   47

Yates' correction   75